Dr Timothy Sharp is a psychologist with an impressive record as an academic, clinician and coach. He runs one of Sydney's most respected clinical psychology practices, a highly regarded executive coaching practice and is the founder of The Happiness Institute, Australia's first and largest organisation devoted solely to enhancing happiness in individuals, families and organisations.

He is Adjunct Professor (in Positive Psychology) within the School of Management, Faculty of Business at the University of Technology Sydney and also an Adjunct Professor (Positive Psychology) within the School of Health Sciences at RMIT University.

As well as being a best-selling author, Dr Sharp is a sought-after public speaker.

www.thehappinessinstitute.com

LIVE HAPPIER LIVE LONGER

Dr Timothy Sharp

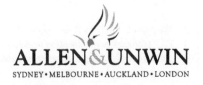

ALLEN&UNWIN
SYDNEY • MELBOURNE • AUCKLAND • LONDON

Published by Allen & Unwin in 2014

Allen & Unwin
Sydney, Melbourne, Auckland, London

83 Alexander Street
Crows Nest NSW 2065
Australia
Phone: (61 2) 8425 0100
Fax: (61 2) 9906 2218
Email: info@allenandunwin.com
Web: www.allenandunwin.com

Cataloguing-in-Publication details are available
from the National Library of Australia
trove.nla.gov.au

ISBN 978 1 74331 918 5

Text design by Melissa Keogh
Set in 11.75/16 pt Birka by Bookhouse, Sydney
Printed and bound in Australia by Griffin Press

10 9 8 7 6 5 4 3 2 1

CONTENTS

'God gave us the gift of life; it is up to us to give ourselves
the gift of living well.'

VOLTAIRE

I've dedicated all of my previous books to my wonderful wife and my two beautiful children.

At the risk of being obvious, however, I'd like to dedicate this publication to my parents, my parents-in-law and the memory of my grandparents. They have all, in different ways, provided me with support, inspiration and wisdom and they've all been great examples of how age need not be a barrier to continuing to live a physically, mentally and socially active life, not to mention one that's meaningful and fulfilling.

In addition, I'd like to make special mention of all the wonderful and inspirational people who agreed to be interviewed for this book. Their stories have added so much colour and flavour, and I'm extremely grateful to them for sharing their experiences, expertise and sagacity.

Thank you so much to all of you; and keep living well!

AUTHOR'S NOTE

In *Anna Karenina*, Tolstoy famously observed, 'All happy families are alike; each unhappy family is unhappy in its own way.'

I'd like to borrow and modify this and write that: All young people are alike: each old person is old in his or her own way.

This book is about what makes some older people significantly healthier and happier than others; it's about how you too can be healthier and happier, regardless of age; and this book is also about how you can help your loved ones to be healthier and happier as they age.

THE BIT BEFORE CHAPTER ONE

'It takes a long time to be young.'
PICASSO

Obviously, I don't know you or the specifics of your life. But there's a good chance that you've been given a gift—a gift that most likely is sitting unwrapped and unaccepted, probably even unrecognised and unacknowledged. A gift that most of us (and much of our culture) have not come to terms with, have not properly integrated into our thinking and not fully (or in many cases even partially) taken advantage of.

The gift is twenty to thirty years of life—another entire adult lifetime—because that's the extra number of years you'll probably live longer than your predecessors, only two or three generations ago. Some have referred to this as the 'longevity revolution', and this evolutionary improvement in life expectancy is a gift we should all be treasuring not ignoring, anticipating with excitement not fear. It's the gift of a 'third age' because, properly enjoyed, this phase of life need not be one of illness or decline but rather, for the vast majority of us, one of growth, wisdom, maturity and more.

Why does this seem like such a radical concept? Why does it seem so at odds with our general view of ageing? Because many of us base our understanding of ageing on the universal concept of entropy—the natural tendency for the universe and everything it contains to fall apart, to decline into chaos.

Yet although this may well apply in many areas of science and specifically physics there's a strong argument to be made that it definitely doesn't apply (or at least that it doesn't *have* to apply) to many aspects of ageing—notably, to those parts of our lives and of our physical beings that grow and improve over time, rather than decline and diminish.

What are these areas that advance and expand? Well, the gaining of wisdom, maturity, and sophistication and the enduring strength of the human spirit. These attributes, and so many others, can contribute to and provide the core components to positive ageing and this gift of the third age. These qualities are ones we all possess but ones whose benefits we may only enjoy once we have acknowledged their existence and actively decided to take responsibility for them.

And this is what this book is about; taking positive action and making positive plans to unwrap and accept the gift we've been lucky enough to have been given. Because as the old saying goes, 'If you fail to plan, you're planning to fail' –and failing in this scenario has some pretty serious consequences.

•

Just over twenty years ago, in 1992, Australia's Prime Minister of the day, Paul Keating, and his Labor government introduced a compulsory 'Superannuation Guarantee' system as part of a major reform package addressing Australia's retirement income policies. This was in response to estimates that Australia, like many other Western countries, would experience a major demographic shift over the next few decades, resulting in the anticipated increase in age pension payments and their placing an unaffordable strain on the Australian economy.

Although a range of advisors from various backgrounds had been providing advice for several decades, the professionalising of and requirement for registration of financial planners was (and remains) a relatively new phenomenon. The introduction of the Financial Services Reform Act of 2001 means most people date the birth of the modern financial planning industry in Australia to 2002. In the decade since then the industry surrounding the provision of financial advice has grown enormously.

The combination of both these unarguably significant events has meant that increasingly Australians are effectively planning and setting themselves up for retirement—but only if you define planning in a purely financial sense, which is mostly what has been done to date.

Now although it is, by no means, a bad thing to plan financially for one's latter years it is vitally important to note that there are other aspects of life for which one should also plan. Few would argue, for example, with the fact that no amount of money will make for a good retirement or a flourishing old age if one's health and happiness is poor.

Which is where this book comes in, because it's worth noting that the gift of the third age is not a monetary gift.

Having worked with one of Australia's largest providers of financial planning advice I have been very impressed by the quality and dedication of many of the industry's professionals. But even they note that in addition to budgeting, saving and wealth creation, there is a range of other issues that will determine the quality of our later years. The better planners ask their clients not just how much money they want in the bank but also how they want to live their lives with that money, and the best planners know that this touches upon issues of health and wellbeing, identity and purpose, relationships and so much more in addition to financial wealth.

The reality is, however, that even the most passionate and enthusiastic financial planners have limited time and not necessarily the expertise with which to help people in these broader areas, which is why I am so excited to be writing this book. My aim is to assist them, their clients, and the many, many others (such as health professionals, carers and family members) who believe as I do that although it is important to plan financially it is equally important—if not more so—to make plans in other areas of our lives; we need to invest in our psychological wellbeing, physical health and interpersonal relationships, for example, as well as those other 'big', less tangible, aspects of life, like its meaning to us as individuals and the concept of spirituality.

In the year before the turn of the century, the United Nations General Assembly decided to declare 1999 as the International Year of Older Persons. Its 'Proclamation on Ageing' was meant to draw attention to the fact that the world's population was rapidly ageing and that with this came enormous challenges and opportunities. However, it does not appear as though much has really changed in the intervening years, despite celebrating ageing through many events and high-profile activities during that year.

As I'll outline in this book, discrimination against older people is rife; myths and misconceptions about ageing dominate popular media and general conversation. Little if anything is being done to educate the massive proportion of our population for whom this is already relevant—or for whom it will soon become relevant—about what they can do to set themselves up for a better and healthier latter life.

And this is all despite the fact that the evidence is there. Good quality scientific research—not to mention a rapidly growing number of wonderfully positive role models with myriad motivational anecdotes—exists to show us the way and provide us with practical strategies we can all use to improve the quality (and length) of our lives.

So if you want to do more than just plan for the financial aspects of your future and to make positive ageing a reality, then take this book to the counter of the store and buy it; click 'check out' online and download it; or, if you've already done one of these, then I'll say thank you very much and carry on reading.

CHAPTER 1

THE PSYCHOLOGY OF POSSIBILITY

'Add life to your days, not days to your life.'
UNKNOWN

Although I love this quote I like to replace the 'not' with an 'and' so it reads, 'Add life to your days *and* days to your life.' Because it's the life you add to your days that adds the days to your life.

Many, many years ago, well before I'd ever considered the idea that eventually became this book, I remember stumbling upon this apocryphal but nevertheless inspirational story:

The 92-year-old petite, well-poised and proud lady, who is fully dressed each morning by eight o'clock, with her hair fashionably coiffed and make-up perfectly applied, even though she is legally blind, moved to a nursing home today.

Her husband of 70 years recently passed away, making the move necessary. After many hours of waiting patiently in the lobby of the nursing home, she smiled sweetly when told her room was ready.

As she manoeuvred her walker to the elevator, I provided a visual description of her tiny room, including the eyelet sheets that had been hung at her window.

'I love it,' she stated with the enthusiasm of an eight-year-old, having just been presented with a new puppy.

'Mrs Jones, you haven't seen the room—just wait.'

'That doesn't have anything to do with it,' she replied. 'Happiness is something you decide on ahead of time. Whether I like my room or not doesn't depend on how the furniture is arranged, it's how I arrange my mind. I already decided to love it. It's a decision I make every morning when I wake up. I have a choice; I can spend the day in bed recounting the difficulty I have with the parts of my body that no longer work, or get out of bed and be thankful for the ones that do. Each day is a gift, and as long as my eyes open I'll focus on the new day and all the happy memories I've stored away, just for this time in my life.'

She went on to explain, 'Old age is like a bank account; you withdraw from what you've put in. So, my advice to you would be to deposit a lot of happiness in the bank account of memories. Thank you for your part in filling my memory bank. I am still depositing.'

And with a smile, she said:

'Remember the five simple rules to be happy: one—free your heart from hatred; two—free your mind from worries; three—live simply; four—give more; five—expect less.'

Regardless of the authenticity of this enchanting, simple story, the idea that ageing in years need not be directly linked to psychological or even physical misery is one that is important and is supported by scientific evidence.

On the one hand there are widely available 'miracle cures'

touted as solutions to the problem of ageing as, for some scientists and theorists, ageing is a 'disease' that's simply awaiting a cure.

The flip side of this idea—that we can halt the effects of ageing—is the assumption that ageing is simply an inevitable process that we need to accept; the level at which we are able to function and perform, both physically and mentally, will decline. Many (if not most) doctors and scientists would say that our cells eventually reach a point where they can no longer divide and so they either die or reach senescence (retirement phase). This is often referred to as the Hayflick limit (named after molecular biologist Leonard Hayflick, who advanced the idea of limited somatic cell division), which argues that no one can live beyond about 120 years.

However, an increasing number of people are starting to believe that this might not be entirely true; that the limits to longevity we've previously considered might not be so concrete. These people argue that the evidence is growing to support the notion that ageing is not an immutable process but rather one that might be amenable to change, either through drug treatments, lifestyle adaptations or both.

Some of this has already been seen—the average life expectancy in Australia, for example, has increased from about 47 years in 1900 to about 82 in 2012. And, impressively, we've not just seen longevity increase but also quality of life. (No one would really want to see people living longer if they were simply extending a period of time in which those people were frail and unwell.)

Although most of this increase in life expectancy has come about due to medical improvements (especially reductions in child mortality), much can be attributed to improved diet and other lifestyle changes. It's also exciting to think of some of the fields of research being explored by scientists (including molecular and cellular repair, hormone and gene therapy) to further lifespan.

Admittedly, some of those claims about extending life are scientifically questionable, but one area of research that's recently received a good amount of attention, and from those considered reputable and respectable, is that looking into telomeres, or the "'end parts' at the tips of our chromosomes", as Fairfax journalist Amy Klein described them in the *Sydney Morning Herald* in 2013. She went on to explain that they serve 'as protective caps for preserving genetic information; think of them as acting like the plastic sheaths that prevent fraying at the ends of shoelaces. The telomeres are disposable buffers blocking the ends of the chromosomes. Without them, genomes would lose information after cell division. A cell's age can be measured by the length of its telomeres.'

Klein noted that in 2009 the Nobel Prize in Physiology or Medicine was awarded to Elizabeth Blackburn, Carol Greider and Jack Szostak for their 1984 discovery of 'how chromosomes are protected by telomeres and the enzyme telomerase'. (Telomerase is a protein that stabilises telomeres when they get worn, causing them to lengthen, and aids cell division.)

At almost exactly the same time another team at the Longevity Genes Project (from the Institute for Ageing Research at the Albert Einstein College of Medicine in New York) discovered a correlation between living to 100 and the inheritance of a mutant gene that makes the human telomerase-producing system extra active and able to maintain telomere length more effectively. For the most part, the people in the study were spared age-related diseases such as cardiovascular disease and diabetes, which together cause the most deaths among elderly people.

What does all this mean?

Well, it means that one of the keys to extending life (and, at the same time, minimising what have traditionally been considered age-related illnesses) is gaining control of the telomere's 'on-off' switch. Although some studies have already achieved limited success with this, there's still a long way to go.

In the meantime, therefore, it's worth looking at other options for promoting longevity because regardless of advances made in genetic engineering (or indeed other, related, fields of medicine and science), according to those at the Human Genome Project genetic factors account for only about 30 per cent of what happens to us—which means that about 70 per cent is determined by lifestyle and/or the environment in which we live.

As exciting as these medical discoveries might seem, the resultant development of medications to prolong life is, in reality, years away. If such drugs do eventually prove to be feasible and affordable, and if they can be delivered without significant side effects (which is always an important question to ask and unfortunately, as history would suggest, a big 'if') then I would be more than happy to queue up for the potion or pill. But what's just as exciting, if not even more so, is that there's also evidence pointing to other interventions that may prolong life and which are within our reach right now!

Through the latter half of the 1970s Ellen Langer, along with a number of colleagues, conducted what has come to be recognised as one of the most significant series of research studies into health and wellbeing. These studies and their far-reaching implications warrant much more attention than they've received to date (outside of academic circles).

In short, Langer's first project focused on the effects of personal responsibility in a group of nursing home residents. One group was simply encouraged to find as many ways as possible to make more decisions for themselves. They were allowed, for example, to choose whether or not to watch movies (and, if they opted to do so, what they watched), where and when to receive visitors and each resident also chose a plant to look after, determining where to place it and when and how much to water it.

A second (comparison) group was simply given the houseplants but advised that the nursing staff would take care of them.

Sounds pretty simple, right? But consider these findings when the residents were followed up eighteen months later.

The members of the first group (those given more personal responsibility) were assessed as being happier and more active. Based on a series of tests given before and after the intervention they were also found to be significantly more mentally alert.

Mindful that both these groups were, to begin with, relatively old and frail, the results become even more interesting. Assessed on several measures, the researchers found that the 'responsibility group' were not only much healthier than the control group, which was what they had expected, but also fewer than half as many of them died during the course of the study than those in the control group!

Just reflect on that for a moment or two—it seems that taking responsibility, even for ostensibly minor decisions such as watering a plant and watching a movie, can make you happier, healthier and (here's possibly the most amazing finding) less likely to die!

In summary then, Langer concluded that due to the power of making decisions and the associated increase in perception of control, residents in the nursing home became healthier and happier, more active and more alert and they ultimately lived longer. Regardless of how you look at it these were (and remain) pretty incredible findings.

But this is not the end of the story. Several years later Langer went on to further explore the ageing process. Taking a slightly different approach this time, she wanted to investigate the possibilities of 'turning back the clock'. In what came to be known as the 'Counterclockwise Study', she devised an ingenious research trial exploring whether recreating a world from an earlier time and inviting a group of people to live in that environment as if it were the present time would impact upon their psychological and physical states.

The experimenters recreated the year 1959, including totally redesigning the furnishings and decorations within a house, in which a number of participants were asked to immerse themselves for a period of time. For all intents and purposes they would be living not in 1979 but in 1959.

In simple terms, Langer has subsequently reflected, the question being asked was, 'If we put the mind back twenty years, would [will] the body reflect this change?'

Another way of framing this question might be: How powerful, really, can the mind be?

According to the results of this study the answer, in short, is 'very powerful'! But let's start at the beginning.

To ensure the study was valid and that the most appropriate variables were being measured, a number of leading experts were consulted about psychological and biological 'markers' of age. After extensive consultation it was determined that the following list of variables would be measured before and after the intervention:

- weight
- dexterity
- flexibility
- vision
- sensitivity to taste
- IQ
- cognitive processing
- memory
- appearance
- self-evaluation.

Then came the task of recruiting volunteers and as is almost always the case in psychological research, the true reasons behind the study needed to be (at least partially) concealed.

Advertisements were placed in the local newspapers inviting people to participate in a project on reminiscing, where individuals in their seventies would spend a week living in a country retreat talking about their pasts. Those who were selected, based on an initial telephone interview, were then invited to a face-to-face meeting to complete the initial psychological and physical tests.

Reading back over the original study, and the experimenters' notes about their experiences, the interviews with the prospective subjects were both interesting and slightly concerning.

Most interviewees listed, extensively, their limitations and the problems they currently experienced. They cited loss of hearing and sight, and most reported multiple activities and hobbies they'd given up due to ill health and/or lack of energy. Sadly, too, many of their (adult) children also spoke of their parents in tones of hopelessness and helplessness and, in some cases, rather derogatory and condescending ways.

The researchers began to question their chances of achieving anything positive with this seemingly decrepit group of old men! Having come this far, though, they reasoned that, at worst, they'd do no harm and that the participants would at least have an enjoyable time for the week, so they persevered and divided the successful candidates into two groups.

Both groups spent a week in the house that had been especially retrofitted to resemble, as closely as possible, a house in 1959 (which was, as noted previously, twenty years earlier). The first or 'experimental' group would reside in the house and would be advised to live as though 1959 were the present time. Everything would occur in the present tense; every conversation, every discussion; life would be lived in 1959 including the ingredients in every meal, the movies watched, and even the magazines and books read. No conversation could mention anything that occurred after 1959 and 'last year' now meant 1958. Finally, all members of this group were asked to write a short autobiography of themselves as though it were 1959 and to bring with them photos of their younger selves (which were then sent to the other house members).

The second or 'control' group lived in the same house, a week later, but was differentiated from the first group in just a few (relatively minor but potentially profound) ways. Firstly, they were asked to write their autobiographies in the past tense; they were asked to bring pictures of their current selves; and once in the house they were invited to reminisce about 1959 as though it was the past (which obviously it was!) rather than consider it as the present day (as the first group were instructed to do).

Before reviewing the results, it's worth noting that considerable attention was given to ensuring everything in the house was an accurate reflection of life in 1959, including details of political and social issues (e.g. the launch of the first US satellite and Fidel Castro's advance into Havana), books, TV and radio programs (including Ian Fleming's *Goldfinger* and *The Ed Sullivan Show*) and furnishings and household objects.

And so I guess you're now wondering how they all fared?

Positive changes in behaviour and attitude were observed almost immediately. In contrast to the old and dependent men who'd entered the house after years of feeling incapacitated and in some cases useless, within days everyone was contributing to the cooking and cleaning up after meals, and almost all of them were functioning far more independently than they had been only days earlier.

Remarkably, when the same tests each participant had completed before the week's house stay were repeated after the completion of the experiment, significant changes were noted. Both groups reported enjoying a fantastic week but notably they were also found to have experienced improvements in hearing, memory and grip strength. Further, the experimental group showed improvements in flexibility, finger length (which indicated improvements in arthritis) and manual dexterity. Sixty-three per cent of the experimental group showed improvements in IQ (as did 44 per cent of the control group); and improvements were also seen in height, gait and posture.

Although both groups' functioning therefore improved significantly, this was in evidence to a far greater extent in the experimental group. These positive changes were interpreted as signs that the participants had got 'younger'—and all this occurred in just one week in an incredible demonstration of the power of the mind and, in the words of the lead author, the 'psychology of possibility'.

The implications of this research go beyond just helping ageing people feel younger and healthier, though. These findings are relevant to us all because they indicate that we can, if we think about our current behaviour and do the right things, live fuller and more satisfying lives at any stage of life. With a helpful attitude, a focus on personal responsibility and a balance between independent functioning and mutual respect we could all achieve so much more than we probably realise.

I'd also like to proffer the notion that we shouldn't wait until we're 70 (or 60 or even 50) years old before beginning to apply these principles (and the many other tools and strategies I'll summarise and outline in this book). Rather, if we start planning and preparing for positive ageing in our thirties and forties we'll be in a much better position to live long and live well.

Indeed, this notion is what this book is all about; this book is for those of you who want to live a full and satisfying life, and a life in which you will continue to thrive and flourish for as long as possible. As Ellen Langer's research suggests, we don't have to deteriorate just because our age has hit a certain number—and even if we have begun to deteriorate it's possible that some of that damage can be reversed!

Accordingly, this book sets out to explain what else we've learned since this 1979 study and what we can do to maximise our chances of living a healthy, happy and long life. I hope that through reading this you'll gain a greater understanding of what we know about health and wellness and, notably, what you can practicably do to keep living well.

And this, at least in part, means reviewing what we consider to be inevitable as we grow older and as we age. One aspect of ageing that (quite rightly and for obvious reasons) always makes the list of inevitabilities is 'death'. Along with taxes, it's unavoidable. Unless I've missed a whole body of research and unless I'm seriously mistaken, we can't stop dying; what we can do, however, is make the most of living. And where we all have choice is in *how* we live.

The good news is that, as briefly referred to earlier, although there's been talk for many years about pills and potions that will extend our years the reality is that there's more scientific evidence supporting the benefits associated with lifestyle changes—things we can all do, changes each and every one of us can make each and every day—to ensure we thrive and flourish into our older years.

This doesn't really surprise me at all because I know several people who live very much like this—and you probably do too. I have a friend, for example, who is 50 years old. Now this might not be considered by you (or many) to be 'old' but the point I want to make here is that most people who meet him typically think he's about 40 (or sometimes even younger).

Why?

Well, because he goes to the gym five or six times each and every week; he keeps his mind stimulated and active by continually reading and learning new things; he eats well (and not too much); he continues to engage in hobbies that he enjoyed when younger (including listening to new and varied music rather than just 'classic hits' or 'golden oldies', trying new restaurants, visiting new places) and although this might appear somewhat superficial, he dresses appropriately but fashionably (which is important for him because it helps him to feel young).

Amazingly, these are the sorts of things that the oldest people in the world also do (although there's not really much research on the dressing bit!), as proved by several studies and surveys on a couple of now-famous populations that have high proportions of older people and centenarians. One of these is on an island in Japan, an island that has come to be known as the Holy Grail of research into positive ageing and longevity, to the extent that it's even been referred to as 'the land of immortals'.

Visiting or even reading about Okinawa is like experiencing a Shangri-La, utopian existence. Despite being invaded, on multiple occasions, by both the Chinese and Japanese, and having its population decimated, Okinawa is where a number of the world's oldest people live.

And live they do. Compared to almost anywhere else in the world they have lower levels of cancer, heart disease and dementia. People who live there just don't seem to age! They continue to live happy, healthy and fulfilling lives way beyond those seen in many other parts of the world and when they do start to look 'old' it's because they're well into their nineties or older, rather than, as seen in many Western cities, their fifties or sixties.

So what's the secret?

A number of people have studied the island of Okinawa and its marvellous inhabitants, including Dan Buettner, who originally worked for *National Geographic* and then went on to speak and write widely on how to live longer.

Buettner isolated at least four key variables or behaviours to which he attributed much of the Okinawans' health and longevity:

1. Diet: the islanders practise what they call *hara hachi bu*, which has been translated as a form of conscious and mindful calorie restriction. That is, they limit what they eat and they remind themselves of this before each and every meal by repeating those words that simply mean: eat until you're 80 per cent full.

2. Activity: the Okinawans spend a lot of time gardening—something that probably has a dual benefit. Because they grow most of their own vegetables and herbs they eat a diet that's high in plant-based foods and that's rich in vitamins, minerals and antioxidants. In addition, they maintain high levels of activity even into old age. Okinawans don't go to the gym (and I've definitely never seen any pictures of them wearing Lycra!) but they keep fit and healthy by farming their land and growing natural, nutritious foods.

3. Optimism: the Okinawans have also been observed to maintain a positive outlook on life. They refer to living for their *ikigai* or what we would probably call a purpose. That is, they know why they get up and out of bed each and every morning and they keep this front of mind each and every day.

4. Connectedness: every Okinawan belongs to a *maoi*, or what we would call a social support group. These groups of peers meet regularly and help each other through the ups and downs of

life, across the whole of their lifespan. You've probably heard the saying, 'It takes a village to raise a child'; well, it could be said that in Okinawa they believe it also takes a village to care for every person.

Enlightening though this information is, none of it is really 'secret' because these behaviours can be seen in several other communities around the world. Dan Buettner identified several others in addition to the most famous and impressive island of Okinawa, referring to these hot spots of longevity as 'Blue Zones'.

Another secluded island, Sardinia (which sits in the Mediterranean off the coast of Italy), is home to the world's oldest living men. This small population includes nearly ten times the number of centenarians (proportionally) as that of the USA.

Historically, the quite rugged landscape of the island has been a home to and workplace of mostly farmers and shepherds. In a remarkable similarity to Okinawa, Sardinia has also been invaded and exploited many times but this ultimately led to what could be considered a health advantage as its inhabitants developed intensely close families and a powerful sense of community.

In the same way as he'd done with the Japanese island population, Buettner identified a number of key behavioural differences that set the Sardinians apart from the broader population and to which he attributed their long lives:

- Gratitude: the Sardinians actively take time, each and every day, to appreciate the beauty of their lives and of their surroundings.
- Respect: they respect their elders and have been observed to nurture very close relationships with their families.

- Humour: they laugh frequently and also tend to have a healthy sense of how humour and perspective can help manage stress and adversity.
- Diet: like the Okinawans, Sardinians eat a diet high in anti-oxidants and anti-inflammatories, with virtually no processed foods.
- Activity: they walk—a lot! Whereas some Westerners seem to associate health and fitness with leaving their desks and sedentary jobs to spend an hour or so in the gym, running a few marathons each year or competing in a corporate triathlon or two, the Sardinians are active almost all day, every day; it's just part of their lives.

Buettner also identified Blue Zones in California, Greece and Costa Rica and, not all that surprisingly, found similarities in the way their inhabitants lived their lives. In addition to those behaviours already noted, he found that the communities with high proportions of healthy, ageing people also practised the following:

- living relatively simple lives with minimal focus on material possessions and maximal focus on relationships and other people in the community;
- prioritising time for calming and relaxing activities and accordingly, experiencing significantly less stress and anxiety than that seen in other populations;
- being altruistic and generous, prizing volunteering. Helping others was par for the course and something that was expected and rewarded within these groups of people.

Again, it's notable that these groups of people have several things in common and each of these have been studied so we can see not only what they do that's different, but also how to put such behaviour into practice ourselves so that the rest of us can enjoy the benefits as well.

How do the people in these Blue Zones live such long and healthy lives? Well, in summary, they:

- have a life purpose, a reason for living and for getting up each and every day;
- respect others and value close familial and community ties;
- foster optimism and a positive attitude for life, laughing often and using perspective to manage stress;
- avoid overeating and consume a diet that's high in plant-based, natural produce with small amounts of protein and 'good fats';
- keep active through the normal course of daily living;
- live a relatively simple life, with health, wellbeing and relation-ships taking precedence over the accumulation of wealth and/or material possessions;
- ensure adequate sleep and rest, typically benefiting from at least eight or nine hours of sleep each night and, in some communities, also enjoying naps during the day;
- think of others, recognising that happiness isn't just about feeling good but also about doing good;
- practise gratitude and appreciation, focusing more on what they have and less on what they don't have;
- respect the older generation. In none of these communities were older people considered frail, weak or incompetent. In fact, quite the opposite was observed as the elders were given greater

respect because of their experience and wisdom (something that unfortunately is not as common in other communities around the world).

The good news is that these are all things each and every one of us can do too. You don't have to move to Okinawa, Sardinia or anywhere else, because the things that the residents of Blue Zones do don't depend on where they live, but on *how* they live.

Take the world's oldest person (at the time of writing this book), for example. Jiroemon Kimura was not from Okinawa but he was from Japan and he lived to be 116 years of age! Just over a year before he died he explained, in an interview, how he lived his life and provided ten tips for others wishing to emulate him:

1. Exercise every day. (Even when his legs began to grow weak, well into his hundreds, Kimura still did 100 bicycle motions, lying on his back in bed, every day.)
2. Eat small portions.
3. Use adversity to grow strong. (No matter how hard things got, Kimura said he faced difficulties with 'endurance and perseverance'. He told people to never let worry or suffering consume them because 'after every storm, peace always comes.')
4. Read and exercise your brain.
5. Eliminate strong preferences and 'take life as it comes'.
6. Live without attachment.
7. Spend time in and with nature.
8. Be grateful and appreciative.
9. Laugh often.
10. Break life up into small, manageable chunks.

If any of these pieces of advice sound familiar it's because they're very similar to the list that I compiled when summarising Dan Buettner's research and the lessons he learned from his Blue Zones.

The point I would like to make again—and again and again and again!—is that none of these behaviours are dependent on living in Japan or Italy or anywhere else special; they are dependent only on a willingness to prioritise health and wellbeing and, therefore, the health- and wellness-boosting activities and attitudes I'll continue to describe throughout this book.

CHAPTER ONE AND A HALF

'You are never too old to set another goal or to
dream a new dream.'
C.S. LEWIS

Following on from the quote above, 'You are never too young to start thinking about positive ageing and preventing the development of possible problems such as dementia,' according to researchers from the Centre for Healthy Brain Ageing (CHeBA) at the University of New South Wales.

In an interview published in *Daily Life*, clinical neuropsychologist Nicola Gates was quoted as saying, 'Dementia might not take hold until later in life but the accumulated insults to the brain that can contribute to its onset can begin decades before.' She went on to state that she believes we need a loud message about maintaining brain health that targets people long before they reach their sixties. 'People don't realise they can start influencing how well their brain ages from a young age—it's time we took a whole-of-life-span approach to preventing dementia.'

Before moving on to the next chapter then, it's worth noting that when I've spoken to and read about those people who continue to thrive and flourish well into their older years, I've discovered that they all live their lives in much the same way, engaging in many of the same sorts of behaviours, for many, many decades. And they don't stop when they reach 40, 50, 60 or even 70!

According to a beautiful profile piece, published in the *New York Times* in September 2013, Harry Rosen is 103 and continues to enjoy many of the simple pleasures he enjoyed pretty much all his working life. For example, Harry eats out at some of New York's finest restaurants every night of the week. And—just in case you've forgotten—he's 103 years old.

As Harry tells it, he entertained quite a lot as part of his business but he determined, when he retired and even after his wife of 70 years died five years prior to the interview, that he would continue engaging in the behaviour that provided him with so much happiness and pleasure.

'It's my therapy, it lifts my spirits . . . it gives me energy', he's quoted as saying. And after the previous chapter on the psychology of possibility, we should not be surprised by this, because Harry is, in many ways, a living, breathing embodiment of the counterclockwise research: he continues to think young and so he feels and lives young.

It's important to add that people like Harry don't just begin their healthy and positive lifestyles at 70, hoping at that point to enjoy another ten to twenty years of good health and wellbeing, but rather they live most of their lives in ways that set them up well for a thriving third age. They actively search for and create, select and store the ingredients that will become their own, very special gift to themselves.

Now obviously we can't go back in time so if you're reading this and thinking that you've not lived most of your life in a way that might set you up for health and happiness then that's not necessarily a problem and you've not necessarily missed the boat because, as the saying goes, 'better late than never'. Anything you start now will still be helpful; any changes you make today will still improve your tomorrow.

So keep reading and keep learning about what the luminaries of positive ageing have done and have achieved and then, quite simply, do whatever makes sense to you and whatever you can to benefit from their experiences and from the associated research.

CHAPTER 2
REDEFINING AGE

'Forget the midlife crisis, this is a midlife opportunity.'

As a father of two children, one a teenager and the other soon to hit adolescence, I've noticed how, over time, what makes my son and my daughter happy has changed. In the early years, happiness or unhappiness essentially came down to food and/or sleep and/or a lack thereof. Toys and stimulation then became paramount only to be replaced, pretty quickly, by sports, dancing and, increasingly, friendships.

Reflecting on this, I've come to learn that what makes any of us happy and what keeps any of us healthy continues to change, not just through adolescence and early adulthood but indefinitely throughout our lives. In hindsight this seems fairly obvious but like many people I'd not given the issue much thought at all until I began to think more seriously about ageing, when researching and writing this book.

And now I invite you to pause and think about what ageing really means, for you and for those around you, and how your needs and desires and hopes and dreams change over time. Because they do change and they should change.

Imagine a 50-year-old pursuing exactly the same pleasures and pastimes as a fifteen-year-old; imagine a 60-year-old who still enjoys the same forms of entertainment as a sixteen-year-old. It is possible to do this, of course, as there are certain activities that can be continued throughout the course of a long life, but it's just as if not more likely that as we age we'll adjust our private and social behaviours in a way that might be labelled 'age appropriate'.

Sandpits tend to be replaced by playgrounds and then bars and nightclubs make way for cafes and restaurants; ultimately, intense episodes of hedonistic pursuits are, more often than not, relinquished for more sedate attempts to achieve satisfaction.

I'm not suggesting here that older people cannot still have a great time; of course they can (and one of the key objectives of this book is to ensure that more older people do, in fact, have a great time). Nor am I suggesting that with age happiness and pleasure are any less important; on the contrary, they're vitally important. And I'm certainly not suggesting that with age comes a decline into boredom and monotony, but I thought I should mention this common assumption, having stumbled upon a very interesting article in *The Atlantic*. Entitled 'How Happiness Changes With Age', Heidi Grant Halvorson included the provocative subtitle, 'Becoming okay with being boring'.

On reading this I was sure I'd be forced to disagree with the content in the main body of the article—not believing that ageing should be equated to becoming boring or dull or to living a life that's in any way uneventful or unexciting—but on reading through the story I realised there were a number of very important and relevant points raised that would be worthwhile including in this chapter.

Halvorson begins thus:

I'm just shy of 40 years old. I spend most Saturday nights at home in yoga pants, rereading favourite novels or watching old movies, or playing Monopoly Junior with my seven-year-old. (If you think Monopoly is boring, then you haven't tried Monopoly Junior.)

This way of spending my Saturday nights makes me happy. If you went back and told my cooler 20-year-old self about the typical evening that awaits the future her, though, she would be pretty devastated that her life turns out to be so . . . boring. That a Saturday night spent reading a book, not even a new book, qualifies as a great time.

She goes on to note that:

Happiness becomes less the high-energy, totally psyched experience of a teenager partying while his parents are out of town, and more the peaceful, relaxing experience of an overworked mom who's been dreaming of that hot bath all day. The latter isn't less 'happy' than the former, it's a different way of understanding what happiness is.

And this 'different way of understanding what happiness is' has been studied by psychologists who differentiate between 'promotion motivation' and 'prevention motivation'. In the former, our focus is predominately on what we can gain while in the latter, we tend to focus more on keeping things running smoothly without risking the loss of anything.

Researchers from Northwestern University in Chicago published findings that indicated promotion-mindedness is most prevalent among the young, because youth is a time for focusing on our hopes for the future. As we age, however, we're less likely to believe we can do anything or that we will live forever. We become keener to hold on to what we've worked hard to achieve and less keen to lose anything of value.

In another fascinating study, researchers from The University of Pennsylvania (The Wharton School) and Stanford University analysed the expression of emotions (particularly positive emotions such as happiness) from more than twelve million personal blogs! In short, they found that the meaning of happiness was not fixed but rather that it changed, systematically, over the course of a lifetime. To quote the authors:

> Whereas younger people are more likely to associate happiness with excitement, as they get older, they become more likely to associate happiness with peacefulness. This change appears to be driven by a redirection of attention from the future to the present as people age.

As fascinating as I consider these research findings to be, and I hope you also find them of interest, I mention them here for one reason and one reason only: because they are consistent with other published findings from a range of other academics in a range of other contexts, showing that happiness means different things to different people at different times of their lives. It's only a small step from there to make the claim that age also means different things to different people at different times of their lives.

For my teenage daughter, 30 or even twenty seems pretty 'old'. As someone of 'middle age', 80 or 90 seems pretty old to me. But when do people of 60 or 70 or 80 think 'old' starts? Having spoken to hundreds of people during the course of working on this book I think it's extremely important for us all to ask: What does 'old' actually mean?

According to several dictionary definitions it's really just an indication of time lived—for example, 'having lived for a long time' or 'relatively advanced in age'. But this is not how it's used in a general sense; most commonly, the word 'old' brings with it negative connotations. It implies degeneration and loss and failure of abilities.

When referring to people, the word 'old' is also used to cover an extremely broad range of ages and could include anyone from 50 upwards. But if an average 65-year-old man today will live to his mid-eighties and a 65-year-old woman will most likely get pretty close to 90, when is old really old? Extending these questions just a little further, what comes to mind when you think of 80 years of age?

At the time I was writing this book Oliver Sacks, the internationally renowned and respected neurologist and bestselling author (of, among other books, *Awakenings*, which was also adapted into a wonderful film, and *The Man Who Mistook His Wife for a Hat*) turned 80. I know this not because I'm a devoted fan of his (although I have always admired his work) but because he wrote a fantastic article explaining his thoughts and feelings about turning 80 for the *New York Times*. My interest was sparked only a few lines in when, in acknowledging that in reality his life was 'almost over', Sacks wrote, quite simply, 'I often feel that life is about to begin'.

He then went on to explain a fascinating piece of personal and family history:

> My mother was the 16th of 18 children; I was the youngest of her four sons, and almost the youngest of the vast cousinhood on her side of the family. I was always the youngest boy in my class at high school. I have retained this feeling of being the youngest, even though now I am almost the oldest person I know.

Were Sacks's comments illustrating yet again how mindset and attitude affect ageing?

Remember the study I referred to earlier in which the elderly men went to live in a house for a week and everything was made to be just like 1959? Remember the stunning results witnessed in which participants metaphorically 'turned back the clock' and literally improved on a range of physical and psychological variables consistent with becoming younger? Well, Ellen Langer, the lead author of that (and subsequent, related) research conducted the study believing that any positive findings would be significant and meaningful because nothing had been trialled in this area and so any hope would be something upon which more could be built. One aspect of the study she and others (including, notably, Stanford University Professor of Psychology Carol Dweck) built upon was what's come to be known as the 'growth mindset' (referred to earlier as the psychology of possibility). People with a growth mindset believe they can improve and achieve better results by working hard; in contrast, those with a fixed mindset believe things are the way they are.

For example, people with a fixed mindset believe they're born with a certain amount of intelligence, talent, ability, personality and even a happiness level. Our genetic make-up is what it is; and there's little they can do about it.

On the other hand, those with a growth mindset believe they can work to improve their performance on intellectual tasks, they can improve talents and skills, they can change their attitude and accordingly, they can enjoy greater happiness and success if they do what they need to do.

Prior to Langer's groundbreaking research the process of ageing was considered very much as something that was fixed. That is, it involved a process of deterioration that was unavoidable and inevitable. Becoming old was equivalent to becoming weaker, frailer, less capable, more forgetful, and so much more, none of which was positive.

But Langer and many others since have shown that things don't have to be like that. Her findings showed that the ageing process doesn't have to be as fixed as most had previously thought. Further, she was at the forefront of a movement that increasingly highlighted the 'mind-body' connection. In fact she was once quoted as saying, 'wherever you put the mind, the body will follow.'

This might remind you of a similar (possibly even more famous) saying—'you're only as old as you feel.' This directly touches on the idea that age is not just a chronological phenomenon but just as importantly, if not more so, one of mindset.

I know I've already touched on this but it bears repeating because it's so important to the concept of positive ageing and it's been supported by so many different studies, investigating the issue from so many different angles.

Did you know, for example, that women who marry men who are much younger than they are live, on average, much longer? And did you also know that women who marry men who are much older than they are die, on average, much younger? And the same is true for men so it's not just a gender issue.

What this means is our 'health age' is at least partly determined by our mindset that can in turn be at least partly determined by living a life that resembles the life of a different age group. How amazing is that?

And even more support comes from even more studies.

In 2002 Becca Levy and her colleagues published a paper in a highly regarded academic journal with the thought-provoking title 'Longevity increased by positive self-perception of aging.' In short, they found that older individuals with more positive self-perceptions of ageing lived up to 7.5 years longer than those with less positive self-perceptions; and these findings held true even when other variables, such as gender, socio-economic status, loneliness and even physical health factors, were taken into account.

Therefore age need not be tied so directly to falling apart and failing; age need not be so closely associated with illness and weakness; chronological ageing might not be something we can stop but health and wellness ageing are almost certainly more within our control. Too often biological processes have been considered linear and inevitable when in fact they might be substantially amenable to change!

Although Langer's original and key research studies were conducted over 30 years ago the prejudices her findings challenged are, unfortunately, still prevalent.

In 2013, for example, the Australian Human Rights Commission published a research report entitled 'Fact or fiction: Stereotypes of older Australians'. This report, among other things, presents how older people are perceived and portrayed in the media—the copy makes for some disturbing reading. Most often, older people were seen as slow, forgetful, vulnerable, grumpy, poor, frail, sick and lonely. As if that were not enough, then in addition older people were also described as bad, weak, stupid, needy, slow, boring, helpless and tired. Only very occasionally did words such as wise, experienced, happy or kind make an appearance.

From this, for me, at least two questions arise:

1. Are these impressions of older people true?
2. Are these portrayals of older people helpful?

In response to the first question, it's interesting to note that the same study revealed that almost half (47 per cent) of all those surveyed felt such descriptions of older people were 'unfair'. The authors themselves described the media portrayal of older Australians as discriminatory and remarked that it substantially neglected the important positive contribution many older people make in a variety of areas. More than unfair, the research suggests that for a significant proportion of older people their media portrayal is simply not true. Rather than grumpy and irritable, many older people are, in fact, happier. Why? Well, according to a study published in the *Journal of Personality and Social Psychology* in

2013 people tend to get happier as they age due (at least in part) to their ability to more effectively manage negative emotions.

In the study, older adults were less likely than younger adults to feel angry and anxious in their everyday lives, as well as when they were asked to perform a stressful task. In addition, older adults scored higher on a test designed to measure how well participants accept their negative emotions. The researchers call this trait 'acceptance', or a tendency to be in touch with rather than to avoid negative emotions.

Notably, the results of this study were not isolated. In a separate project a professor of psychology from Stony Brook University surveyed more than 300,000 people and also found that a significant number of people became happier as they aged. Whereas the previously referred to research highlighted the acceptance and management of negative emotions as key contributors to an increase in happiness with age, this piece of work hypothesised that this was most likely due to a number of variables, including: a deeper appreciation of the value of life; a feeling of fulfilment; a greater ability to understand and handle life's vicissitudes; fewer (and more realistic) aspirations and expectations; the ability to live in the present and not worry about the future; the wisdom to know we can't please everyone all the time; and an inclination to see situations more positively.

And there's more evidence to this effect. In June 2013 Britain's Office for National Statistics revealed the results of a large-scale survey, involving more than 40,000 households, indicating that retirement makes people feel happier and healthier than they have done at any point since their mid-thirties. The results also found that people in their late sixties feel like they are back in their prime, with similar levels of satisfaction with their health to those 30 years younger. Further, the incidence of anxiety and depression drops by almost a third between the early fifties and late sixties.

Whatever the cause of happiness increasing with age, the point here is that the incredibly negative perceptions of older people referred to earlier, including the common descriptor of 'grumpy', are simply not true in many, many cases.

In *Aging with Grace*, David Snowdon reports findings that 40 per cent of the general population remains 'fully functional' beyond the age of 85. In the famous and much-respected Harvard Grant study (a 75-year examination of human development), slightly different measurement criteria were used but it could easily be concluded from their data that approximately 55 per cent of the men aged between 85 and 90 were living active lives with few or minimal limitations in activities of daily living (such as walking, hiking, moving light furniture, climbing up and down stairs, dressing and personal care).

Similarly, in the very highly regarded *Handbook of Positive Psychology*, Gail Williamson (a Professor of Psychology at the University of Georgia) writes in her chapter about ageing well:

An important truth, albeit persistently denied by much of the population, is that most adults over the age of 65 are remarkably healthy. Rates of disability, even among the very old (i.e., those over 95), are steadily declining. Only 5.2% of older adults live in nursing homes and similar facilities, a drop of 1.1% since 1982. In 1994, 73% of adults 78-84 years of age report *no* disabling conditions, and among the 'oldest old' (i.e., those over age 85), fully 40% had no functional disabilities.

Williamson goes on to paint an even rosier picture, noting that although some cognitive decline is more common in older people, many of the comparisons made in the research were with college students (which is always of questionable validity) and that ageing adults themselves must bear some responsibility, as much of the decline can be attributed to a lack of 'mental exercise' (with people tending to challenge and stimulate themselves much less as they age). The adage 'use it or lose it' is very relevant here: those who make sure they continue to regularly engage in mentally stimulating activities will continue to enjoy higher levels of functioning.

Williamson also puts forward strong arguments against the common beliefs that older people are lonely and isolated, and that accordingly they drain society's resources. She cites research reported on in the Macarthur Foundation Study of Aging in America and findings published by the Center for the Advancement of Health, noting that the functioning of older people is, in general, much better than most believe and that there's little or no evidence that they incur greater costs on society or public resources.

Further, she concludes that advances in medical technology along with improvements in the understanding and treatment of most chronic diseases mean that baby boomers and subsequent generations have much to look forward to.

There is even some positive local data, obtained from research conducted right here in Australia. Published by Associate Professor Michael Coory in the *Medical Journal of Australia*, a paper entitled 'Ageing and healthcare costs in Australia: a case for policy-based evidence?' posits, 'There have been dire predictions that population ageing will result in skyrocketing health costs. However, numerous studies have shown that the effect of population ageing on health expenditure is likely to be small and manageable.'

Coory goes on to argue that these pessimistic predictions have stifled real and meaningful debate, limiting the number of policy options considered, but notes they've been 'popular' because they fit with certain 'ideological positions that favour growth in the private sector and seek to contain health expenditure in the public sector.'

Coory concludes by stating, 'the available evidence indicates that population ageing will only have a limited effect on healthcare costs, and there is no evidence that population ageing will cause chaos for our health system.'

Being unfair and neglectful of the older members of society is one thing; being unhelpful and allowing politics to get in the way of good healthcare decision-making is another.

Following on from this it's not hard to imagine how the aforementioned negative perceptions are unhelpful, especially if one reflects on Ellen Langer's research. The exciting conclusions that many drew from her work—that by adopting a more positive and constructive self-perception older people could enjoy major health benefits—are undermined by the existence of negative self-perceptions, which could easily stem from negative public perceptions (propagated and reinforced by the media and others), which are in turn most likely associated with poor physical health and poor psychological wellbeing.

In short, then, it befits and benefits none of us to talk about older people in a way that's neither true nor helpful. If it contributes to their ill-health and poor psychological status then ultimately, it impacts on all of us because a sick and sorry elderly population (as opposed to a healthy and happy one) will, to put it bluntly, be an expensive burden on the whole of society, unlike a healthier and happier elderly population, which could—and should—be a positive contributor.

However, as an optimist I believe there is always a solution.

And at least part of the solution will come from looking at the facts and using them to redefine ageing. Let's remind ourselves of what we really know about older people:

- According to a United Nations study entitled 'Ageing in the 21st Century: a celebration and a challenge' 47 per cent of males and 24 per cent of females over 60 years old still participate in the labour force; in some developing countries, over 90 per cent of people over 60 work. (There are obviously economic explanations for this, not all of which might be considered positive, but it does reflect that this group of people can be considered, at least in one way, active and functional.)
- According to research from the University of Hawaii, 'illness should not be an expected, and thus an accepted, companion during the later years'. (I.e. the elderly don't have to be sick and frail.)
- In research from a large Gallup poll, in which approximately 340,000 people were surveyed, many older people reported getting happier as they got older.
- A paper published by The Australia Institute in 2004 makes a point of noting that 'an ageing population does not necessarily mean a sicker population burdening the country with large medical and social care costs. In fact, the baby boomer

population is projected to be healthier, more active and more productive than preceding generations'.

- The Australia Institute report also refers to research that points out that although a significant proportion of all lifetime healthcare costs (more than 25 per cent) are incurred in the final year of life the cost of this last year does not increase with age. If anything, it's more likely to fall, as the most costly patients tend to be those who die young!

Not only, therefore, is an older population not necessarily dysfunctional, sicker or more costly than a younger one, but it can actually provide significant benefits for communities and the economy, as shown in the examples below:

- Multiple studies, including at least one conducted by the Australian Institute of Health and Welfare, have found that many organisations and institutions will benefit from the surge in numbers of older people who are active and healthy, independent and who have time on their hands. These people are ready, willing and able to provide volunteer services and will be increasingly in demand because of their experience and dedication.
- Far from being 'net receivers' of help and support, older people are, in fact, 'net providers' through the provision of childcare, financial support and practical as well as emotional assistance to family and friends.

Acknowledging the contributions that can be made by the older members of society, perhaps we need to redefine that word—retirement.

I remember growing up and hearing my grandparents (and their peers) talk about retirement. To be perfectly honest, it sounded fantastic. Discussions included travel and tasting great foods, games of lawn bowls, tennis and golf and essentially having a good time without pressure, responsibility or obligation and that was full of pleasure, rest and relaxation.

My parents (and parents-in-law) are now at the age my grandparents were back then and the life they're living is completely different from the life I imagined an 'older' person would live when I was younger. There are various reasons for this and numerous ways in which my parents' retirement differs from that of my grandparents but, in short, most, if not almost all the people I know over 60 and even over 70 are extremely active.

Look up 'retirement' in a dictionary and you'll find definitions such as these:

- removal or withdrawal from active service, office, or business
- withdrawal into privacy or seclusion
- seclusion from the world
- the act of retreating.

'Retirement' used to essentially mean the cessation of any meaningful or valuable contribution or attempts at productivity.

How things have changed—and for a variety of reasons.

But putting these aside for now, there's no doubt that the way the majority of older people understand retirement in this day and age has substantially changed from their predecessors. It now seems to involve slowing down but not stopping and a prioritisation of leisure but continuation of work. Although some note they can't afford to spend the final few decades of their lives not earning an income most also claim that they wouldn't want to stop working even if they could.

'Boomers reject the notion of a "balloon payment" of leisure stretching out for decades beyond traditional retirement age,' says Marc Freedman, CEO of Encore.org and author of *The Big Shift: Navigating the New Stage Beyond Midlife*. Instead, Freedman sees a trend toward 'encore careers', in which people take up new work at midlife that is personally and socially meaningful, perhaps moving at a slower pace. He regards this as a good thing because there's a considerable amount of research clearly indicating that retiring in the old sense of the word can be bad for one's health!

People who stay in the workforce past traditional retirement age live longer (assuming all other variables are equal), while those who stop working, in contrast, typically see a decline in their mobility and in their mental health. Among other things, these problems can be attributed to less social contact and less cognitive challenge.

Separate studies from Harvard University, the Institute of Economic Affairs in the UK and the US-based National Bureau of Economic Research have all drawn the same conclusions—that there are substantial, negative effects on health after retirement. In slightly different ways each of these studies arrived at the same results, that retirement (as it's traditionally been defined) was associated with a significant increase in clinical depression and a decline in self-assessed health; further, they found that these effects increased with the number of years people spent in retirement. And I can attest to this conclusion, having seen it all with my own eyes.

In my clinical psychology and executive coaching practice I've witnessed, in many cases, sadly, the negative impacts of old-fashioned retirement. I've sat down with clients who've previously lived fulfilling, satisfying and highly productive and successful lives only to find the golden years they were hoping for didn't materialise when they left their jobs or sold their businesses. Many struggled to find meaning in life, to understand who they now were without their occupations or professions and, ultimately, many struggled to replace what they'd lost or given away with anything as pleasurable or satisfying.

And why would this be a surprise? Why would we expect a life without structure, social interaction, meaning, purpose, achievement and accomplishment to be enjoyable?

This is not to say there's no such thing as a happy retirement but as I hope you're starting to see, the new and healthy definition of retirement needs to be one in which several criteria are met and these criteria are effectively the same as those required for healthy ageing.

I need look no further than my own immediate family (all of whom described below are in their early seventies) to give some fabulous examples of healthy and happy ageing and 'retirement':

- My mother plays bridge almost every day of the week. This activity provides her with fantastic cognitive stimulation as well as social interaction (and some physical activity). When not playing bridge she's often helping out with grandchildren.
- My father has for many years been very involved in Rotary International, including a recent stint as District Governor. He's also served on several boards and consults to a number

of charities and organisations in his area of expertise. All of this provides significant physical, mental and social activity that keeps him busy and fulfilled. (My father's current wife continues to be heavily and actively involved in Rotary, which also partially extends my father's activities in this area.)

- My father-in-law plays tennis regularly, monitors a number of investments and assiduously keeps up to date with news and current affairs, all of which keeps him 'sharp as a tack', both physically and mentally.
- My mother-in-law has weekly walk-and-talk sessions with her 'girlfriends' (which covers both the physical and social aspects of healthy living) and she's very active in the care of all of her grandchildren.

I'm not suggesting by any means that my parents and in-laws are in 'perfect health' but there's no doubt that at '70 plus' they're all fabulously active, mentally and physically, and continuing to enjoy and contribute to life in many ways.

So as you read through the remainder of this book, give some thought to your definitions of 'ageing' and 'retirement' and other related constructs. Beware of any unhelpful and unhealthy assumptions about ageing and remember how important your mindset is because it will literally, and directly, impact upon your health and wellbeing and quality of life.

CHAPTER TWO AND A HALF

If, like me, you were brought up being told, 'It's the thought that counts', then I just want to take a minute to partially challenge that belief before we go any further.

Thoughts clearly count, as I'll discuss in much more detail in Chapter Four, but it is just as important, if not more so, to also note that actions speak louder than words.

I hope the previous two chapters have stimulated your thinking and encouraged you to reconceptualise your definitions of ageing and retirement. But I also hope that reading this book is beginning to motivate you to actually change the way you live your life with a view to enhancing its length and quality.

At The Happiness Institute (the positive psychology coaching and consulting practice I established in 2002) we've been saying for well over a decade now that achieving happiness requires nothing more than practising a few simple disciplines each and every day. It would be just as valid to say this about achieving longevity so start putting your thoughts into practice—start doing what healthy ageing people do to start reaping the rewards: enjoyment, life satisfaction, health, wellbeing and more.

CHAPTER 3

PHYSICAL ACTIVITY AND EXERCISE: DIET, SLEEP AND REST

'We don't stop playing because we grow old.
We grow old because we stop playing.'
GEORGE BERNARD SHAW

Several years ago I met Tristan White, a very entrepreneurial health professional who was passionate about what he did and who had established what has become over the last ten years or so one of the most successful physiotherapy practices in this country—The Physio Co, specialising almost exclusively in working with residents of aged care facilities.

In the organisation's words, 'The Physio Co helps oldies stay mobile, safe and happy!' When I spoke to Tristan again recently about this book he explained that, 'it's the things you and I take for granted, that can be lost during ageing, that can take away from a person's happiness.' Things like, he noted, the ability to get in and out of bed, to get to the bathroom and to dress without assistance and to walk to the local shops independently. Although these things might appear to be relatively minor in the general scheme of things they're nevertheless impairments that potentially contribute to a loss of freedom; and there's no doubt that a loss of freedom can contribute to a decline in happiness that can then lead to deficits in health and wellbeing more generally.

Thankfully, all aged care residents are required to undergo a full physiotherapy assessment when newly admitted to an aged care facility in Australia and so Tristan and his team (and, of course others who are performing similar duties) are in a great position to present care plans and make recommendations that ideally will keep these residents active, healthy and happy for as long as possible. All too often, however, he reports that he and his team see problems with lack of mobility, chronic pain, fear of falling and other problems that impact upon the basic tasks of daily living.

As noted earlier, Tristan is passionate about what he does and hopeful for a better future. During our discussion he did not, in any way, seem disillusioned with or despairing about the problems he sees. Rather, he focused on his belief that it doesn't have to be like this.

'It's an old message,' Tristan said when we spoke, 'but one that still rings true. Move it or lose it.'

Which is, if one thinks about it, a very positive message. Because what it means is that if we do keep moving we can keep using—our bodies will keep working for as long as we keep working our bodies.

It's amazing what you see once you begin to become aware of something. Once I started researching and writing this book I began to see, almost everywhere and almost all the time, wonderful examples of healthy ageing and older people living lives that could only be described as fantastic examples for us all to follow.

As a psychologist this shouldn't have been all that surprising to me as I've been aware for many years now, ever since my days as a student, of a well-researched phenomenon referred to as 'priming'. Basically, priming describes the effect we've all experienced of noticing something more once we're aware of it. So if, for example, you buy a new small, white hatchback car, you're markedly more likely to notice lots of small and white hatchback cars. Along similar lines, I distinctly remember when my wife was pregnant that all of a sudden there were pregnant women everywhere; and just a few months later there were babies and prams everywhere.

This phenomenon is relevant because I hope now, having read the previous two chapters, that you'll notice more examples of positive ageing and healthy and happy older people. Accordingly, I hope that new attitude to ageing will directly impact upon your own health and wellbeing, as it can be seen to do in much of the research cited earlier.

Another reason I raised this issue here was that I, along with friends and colleagues, had begun to notice older people achieving impressive physical feats. One in particular stood out; featuring in the *Huffington Post* it was about a 79-year-old woman who'd broken fifteen world records in track and field (which would be impressive for anyone at any age!).

Although she'd played competitive tennis before, Flo Meiler only began track and field when she was 65 (an age when, sadly, many people have given up almost all physical activity let alone competitive sport); and she only decided to give it a shot because the sport needed people desperately. In the fourteen years since becoming an elite athlete she's held not only the fifteen world records mentioned, but also another twelve national records (in the United States). And she's still competing.

This grandmother to five and great-grandmother to two trains six days a week and describes being in 'the best shape I've ever been'. She is, remember, 79 years of age.

Not all that surprisingly she was quoted as saying, 'It's never too late' and, 'You're never too old.' Her strong belief that 'people can still get better as they age' is central to what this book is all about so Meiler could even be seen as my personal ambassador and a hero for the positive ageing movement. But she's not alone. There are many other heroes out there—most unknown to the general media and even, in many cases, to their local communities.

Amazingly, just a day after reading the *Huffington Post* article, my brother contacted me with a suggestion. He's been a very keen and very dedicated long distance runner for many years now (having completed multiple half- and full marathons) and he's a member of a large running group in our home city known as the Sydney Striders. After becoming aware of my latest project he told me that I just *had* to talk to a man by the name of Frank Dearn. 'Frank,' he wrote in an email, 'is a legend of the Striders . . . and quite a character too!'

After such praise, I was pretty keen to have this man tell his story for this book and, thankfully, Frank was more than happy to oblige.

Now 80 years of age, Frank only started running in his forties, mostly in response to the lethargy he was experiencing around the middle of the day when he was working as a solicitor. He went on to complete his first marathon at the age of 65, a time when many of his peers were (literally and metaphorically) hanging up their boots. (When I spoke to Frank he'd just completed yet another marathon, aged 80, only one week before our chat.)

Since he took up the sport, Frank told me, he's completed more than fourteen marathons, multiple half marathons and one of Australia's (if not the world's) toughest distance races, the 45-kilometre Six Foot Track, which takes place in rugged bushland and includes several almost-vertical climbs. He's actually completed this event three times!

But the many awards, accolades and records he's collected over the years mean little if anything to Frank. He runs, he explains, for the camaraderie and for the health benefits. And he's not the only one that benefits from his healthy activity and running exploits. In a story about Frank, published in *Runner's World* magazine, another Sydney Strider, Dale Thomson, explains that Frank is an inspiration to many. 'Frank inspires people in ways he doesn't even know about. He's really just living his life and getting out there and giving it a go, which is something everyone admires.'

What both Flo and Frank illustrate is the importance of physical exercise and regular activity for the positive ageing process. Does age really need to slow us down as much as many of us might have thought? Playing with the quote with which I began this chapter, do we stop exercising because we're growing old or do we grow old because we stop exercising?

Regardless of age we are still all physical beings living in bodies that were designed to be active and to move. (Remember back to the residents of the Blue Zones, especially those in Sardinia and Okinawa.) When we stop this activity and movement our bodies start to deteriorate.

And it's not just about aerobic fitness or muscular strength (although these are undeniably important). Dr John Ratey, an Associate Clinical Professor of Psychiatry at Harvard Medical School, has been quoted as saying, 'Exercise is one of the few ways to counter the process of ag[e]ing because it slows down the natural decline of the stress threshold.'

In reviewing this topic, including much of Dr Ratey's work, Canadian social worker and writer Diana Boufford notes that a lack of (or reduction in) movement can trigger a domino effect. That is, once people stop moving adequately they can begin to experience a range of other, linked health problems, including having trouble walking, standing and getting in and out of chairs; bowel difficulties; as well as practical problems associated with tasks of daily living such as cooking, cleaning, washing, and dressing. These are the sad realities, at the end stages of life, that Tristan White and his team at the Physio Co see each and every day.

The evidence shows that maintaining regular, adequate physical activity can prevent or at the very least significantly delay the onset of such problems—as well as markedly reducing the risk of depression, improving mood and enhancing quality and quantity of sleep.

Amazingly, exercise therapy has even been found to help people with Parkinson's disease. Susan Fox, professor of neurology at the University of Toronto, has written that although it's early days in terms of research in this area, the evidence is mounting. She believes strongly that exercise therapy is emerging as a new and exciting area of treatment for Parkinson's, not only because it can lead to significant improvements in symptoms, but also because it has minimal side effects and comes with a whole lot of additional health benefits.

It's important to clearly state that there's currently no cure for Parkinson's disease, but many drugs are available that help minimise and control its symptoms, mainly by boosting dopamine levels in the brain. According to Professor Fox, 'There's now some preclinical [early] evidence that when patients move and exercise that it releases dopamine within the brain, so there's some biological evidence that it may actually have a positive symptomatic effect.'

Still not convinced about the benefits of exercise? What if I were to tell you that exercise can also help to reduce the risks of developing dementia—because it can!

Dr Nicola Gates is a Sydney-based neuropsychologist (to whom I referred earlier), who believes that although dementia might not become evident and obvious until later in life it's never too early to start actively working on preventing it. She was recently quoted in a *Sydney Morning Herald* article on this topic as saying, 'People don't realise they can start influencing how well their brain ages from a young age—it's time we took a whole-of-lifespan approach to preventing dementia.'

As I'll discuss later, having a healthy diet and maintaining a healthy weight can help with this but so too can other healthy habits, especially participating in regular exercise. In the same article, Perminder Sachdev (co-director at the Centre for Healthy Brain Ageing at the University of New South Wales) was also quoted as saying, 'About half the risk of dementia is related to lifestyle factors . . . exercise may be the most important protective factor for ageing brains. Ideally, it should start early and be maintained into later life, though it's never too late to start.'

'People who exercise have better cognitive function, especially memory and executive function [the brain skills involved in organisation, planning and judgements], and lower dementia risk,' Gates says. 'While our brains shrink with age, there's evidence regular exercise can help counteract this by increasing the numbers of brain cells and the connections between them, along with the extra blood flow needed to sustain this new growth.'

And it doesn't have to be competitive running or athletics in the manner of the two great examples cited earlier (Flo and Frank); remember the Blue Zone communities researched and written about by Dan Buettner? In each and every one of those groups of people, daily activity was a regular, normal and accepted part of life. They might not have been running marathons like Frank, or pole vaulting metres in the air like Flo, but they were farming, cooking (old-style) and walking—moving their bodies each and every day in ways that anyone would consider healthy and helpful. (Just as importantly, it's worth noting what they weren't doing, which was spending hours and hours—most of their days—engaged in sedentary activities such as extensive TV-watching or working on computers.)

And here's some really good news for those of you who don't necessarily like getting all hot and sweaty working out in the gym or running for miles on the road—there are plenty of fun ways to exercise from which all of the same benefits can be redeemed.

In 2003 one of the world's most esteemed medical journals, the *New England Journal of Medicine*, published a fascinating paper entitled 'Leisure activities and the risk of dementia in the elderly'.

As its title suggests, the authors examined the relationship between leisure activities and dementia risk in the elderly, studying almost 500 people aged over 75 who were living in the community and who at the start of the study did not suffer from dementia.

Over the next five years all the subjects were followed up and dementia (of various types) developed in about a third of the group. Interestingly, however, a number of activities were clearly associated with a significantly reduced risk and these activities included reading, playing board games, playing musical instruments and dancing.

Now it should be noted that the greatest effect of these leisure activities was measured in cognitive terms—so if you keep your brain active you're less likely to develop dementia. But what was most interesting, in the context of this chapter, was that dancing also had a substantial positive impact.

Other studies have also sung the praises of dancing, as it is an activity that generates three key clearly beneficial outcomes. As just noted, there are cognitive benefits associated with dancing as the requirement to remember set moves and routines involves using the memory and strategic-thinking parts of the brain quite considerably. In addition, dancing is also typically a social activity and social interaction is one of the best things we can do for our health and wellbeing—at any age (as I'll elaborate upon in Chapter Five). Finally, dancing is (in addition to a cognitive and social activity) a physical activity—it's a form of exercise. And so for those who don't have any desire or intention to run marathons or compete in athletic events, you can join the local dance group or—even more simply—turn on your favourite music, find a friend, and start to boogie!

Running, track and field, dancing—there are so many ways in which you can keep your body fit and healthy and, therefore, extend the length and quality of your life; the number of ways you can 'exercise' is really only limited by your imagination.

To give yet another example, doing housework—although not necessarily considered 'fun'—can be a highly effective form of healthy activity, as long as you think about it the right way.

Consider this fascinating piece of research: 84 female room attendants working in seven different hotels were measured on a number of physiological variables, known to be associated with and affected by physical exercise. Half the women were told that the cleaning work they routinely completed was good exercise and that it satisfied the government body's recommendations for an active lifestyle. The other women were not told anything about the relationship between their work and exercise.

Notably, the behaviour of neither group changed over the course of the experiment. The only 'intervention' was telling some of the workers that what they were already doing was a form of good, healthy activity. Now here comes the interesting part. Firstly, when the participants were followed up four weeks after the study, those in the 'informed' group perceived themselves to be getting significantly more exercise than they had prior to the experiment. And, amazingly, when compared to the other group they showed significant improvements in weight, body fat percentage, hip-to-waist ratio, body mass index and blood pressure. And note again—this was without actually changing their behaviour at all, just changing their perception of their existing behaviour.

The best thing about these research findings is that too often we think we can't exercise because we don't have time. But the reality is, you might not need to find or create more time for 'exercise'; you may well already be engaging in healthy activities which, if just reinterpreted or thought about in a different way (like those in the hotel room attendants' study), could pay greater dividends.

Let's take a minute to get really practical, and consider the range of possible activities anyone could participate in, alongside their respective benefits:

- *Walking*—this is one of my favourite exercises, for anyone of any age, if for no other reason that it can be done by anyone, any time, anywhere. It costs nothing and requires no equipment (although a good, comfortable pair of shoes would be ideal). But importantly, walking has been shown to improve both strength and aerobic fitness.
- *Jogging*—for those willing and able to increase the intensity a bit, jogging or running is also a fantastic form of exercise as, like walking, it can be done anywhere and at any time. And in addition to the more obvious benefits in terms of aerobic fitness jogging has also been shown to also improve memory and cognitive functioning.
- *Tai chi*—this Chinese martial art comprises a series of relatively gentle stretches and poses that flow easily from one position to the next. As a form of exercise it is low-impact and causes minimal stress to joints, nor does it strain the cardiovascular system. But most importantly, it's been shown to improve balance and core strength that can together reduce the risk

of falling. The benefits of reducing the risk of falling are obvious but it's worth explicitly noting here that according to the Centers for Disease Control and Prevention in the United States, falls are the leading cause of injury-related death and the most common cause of non-fatal injuries and hospital trauma admissions among adults aged 65 or older. One in three older people falls every year, resulting in millions of injuries and, sadly, thousands of deaths. That's why it's so important to be able to maintain your balance.

- *Yoga*—similar to tai chi, yoga is a gentle form of exercise and it combines stretching, strengthening and controlled breathing, all of which have fantastic health benefits. Several studies have confirmed this, noting all those achieved by tai chi as well as, among others, improvements in sleep.

- *Squats*—a range of simple exercises can be done at home without the need for expensive or complex machines or equipment. One of the best of these is the good old-fashioned squat. The benefits include keeping the legs strong and stable—something that's important for basic daily tasks like getting up and down or in and out of a chair, and climbing stairs. As noted above, lower-body strength and stability can also reduce the risk of falls, something that becomes all too common if strength is allowed to deteriorate through inactivity.

- *Weightlifting*—just as jogging takes walking to another level of intensity (and, potentially, to another level of benefit), so too can weightlifting provide considerable paybacks to anyone of any age. Most notably, resistance training such as this (performed for about 30 minutes at least three times each week) can prevent bone loss and conditions such as osteoporosis (a condition that in 2008 was estimated to affect more than 600,000 people in Australia). Historically, weight training was seen as a form of exercise that was only appropriate for body builders or narcissistic young men! Increasingly, however, its benefits are being touted for almost everyone of any age as the line between aerobic and anaerobic forms of training becomes blurred.

- *Swimming*—this is yet another fantastic form of exercise for anyone and especially for those who suffer from some form of arthritis. A Canadian study recently showed that regular swimming and hydrotherapy (water-based exercising) significantly reduced people's chances of falling and of breaking bones. Researchers have also claimed that swimming has additional anti-ageing benefits such as easing arthritic pain and increasing flexibility and mobility.

- *Laughter*—let's not forget one of the best forms of exercise and of medicine: laughter (which is in a league of its own when it comes to exercising your internal organs!). Laughter has been shown to provide innumerable physical and psychological benefits—it's a good form of aerobic activity and a powerful mood enhancer.

It can therefore be clearly seen that there are many options for those considering physical activity and exercise—and that is just my shortlist! (I could also have included bike-riding, roller skating, surfing and team sports such as tennis, bowls and soccer). But when it comes to physical health and wellbeing we shouldn't just focus on exercise. Nutrition and diet are also vitally important, as are sleep and rest.

Nutrition and diet

If you remember back to the commonalities that were present across each of those communities with higher than normal proportions of healthy older people and centenarians, it was pretty clear that they also differed from other communities in terms of what and how much they ate. Those who lived longer and better tended to eat a predominantly plant-based diet and they tended to eat less. (Remember the Japanese idea of eating until 80 per cent full?)

Now there are many reasons for this but it should be noted that it's not necessarily a new approach at all. In fact the ancient Greek philosopher, Epicurus, who's wrongly been considered in the past as a hedonist and glutton, advocated several thousand years ago that we must 'learn to be content with what satisfies fundamental needs, while renouncing what is superfluous.'

And modern-day medicine certainly supports this. According to Dr John Ratey, the health academic and expert referred to earlier in the discussion on exercise, 'We are in danger of eating ourselves to death and killing our brains in the process'.

And he's not on his own in holding concerns about this. In an ongoing national program of studies in the United States (the National Health and Nutrition Examination Study or NHNES), the health of 11,145 people (comprising adults and children) was surveyed and the results are very worrying. The research revealed that adults over the age of 60 had higher levels of abdominal obesity and hypertension (abnormally high blood pressure) than any other age group tested, except those 80 years and older, whose levels of abdominal obesity and hypertension were even higher.

The authors of the research study went on to state, 'nutrition plays a significant role in prolonged health and health promotion throughout the life course. Owing to relationships identified between nutritional intake and mild cognitive impairment, depression, physical deterioration, and quality of life, promotion of successful aging in older adults should include healthy dietary practices.'

'Healthy dietary practices' need to include, among other things, moderate eating—or, in other words, not overeating. In short, research conducted in this country, in the eastern suburbs of Sydney, has found that elderly people who overeat are at greater risk of severe brain shrinkage and dementia.

According to one of the researchers, Professor Katherine Samaras of the highly acclaimed Garvan Institute, the findings are a warning to all people, particularly the elderly, to make sure they don't eat more than they need.

Pretty simple really: in order to live a longer, healthier and happier life one needs to be mindful of one's diet.

Before going any further, I should note here that I'm not a qualified dietician or nutritionist and so I'm somewhat reluctant to give specific dietary advice (particularly because everyone is different so advice should be tailored appropriately to suit an individual's specific needs) but I list below the general recommendations provided by Nutrition Australia (experts in this area), a non-government and non-profit peak community nutrition education body, set up to provide scientifically based nutrition information to encourage all Australians to achieve optimal health through food variety and physical activity:

- Use less salt—avoid adding salt to foods and restrict the use of highly salted foods such as corned beef, bacon and luncheon meats and snack foods such as potato chips.
- Drink more water—consume small amounts of water regularly, throughout the day, to ensure you stay hydrated.
- Avoid excessive consumption of other liquids—although perfectly fine for most people in moderation, it's typically advisable to minimise caffeine (coffee and tea), alcohol and especially carbonated soft drinks.
- Eat a diet high in nutrients and vitamins—this can mostly be achieved by eating plenty of plant-based foods such as fresh vegetables and fruits.
- Ensure adequate consumption of calcium—this is important to avoid or reduce loss of mineral content in bones and, in the worst cases, osteoporosis. For most people this can be achieved by including adequate dairy foods in one's diet, such as milk and cheese.
- Avoid gaining weight and/or allowing yourself to become overweight—this will help avoid a range of problems including loss of or limited mobility and, in some cases, arthritis. For most people this usually and quite simple means eating a bit less than they might have done in the past.
- Protein is also important—lean meats are typically the best sources of protein (so supplement the vegetable components of your diet with mostly fish and chicken, and some red meats also) but so too are eggs, tofu, legumes (beans), nuts and seeds.
- Keep the fibre content up—consumption of high-fibre foods is also important to avoid constipation and other gut and digestive problems. So include, in your balanced diet, wholegrain

affected by a range of emotional, psychological and motivational factors, all of which are vitally important to its success.

You can learn more about The Happiness Diet on its dedicated website (see the resources section at the end of this book) but in short, it's based on an idea I developed after spending many years working with people who were trying to find happiness (and who were successful in various different ways). During this time I discovered that one of the main obstacles to happiness (and success) is what I came to call 'the tyranny of when'.

'The tyranny of when' is the phenomenon we've all experienced at some time or other when we say to ourselves (or to others) that 'I'll be happy when . . .' ('. . . I have more money,' '. . . I have a bigger house,' or—and this is the one that I began to hear more and more in our era of global obesity—'I'll be happy when I lose weight.')

The problem for many people is that (for a variety of reasons) they never get there; and even if they do, they then think of something else that they 'need' before they can really feel happy. Bigger houses, bigger mortgages, snazzier cars, the bigger, better super-duper slice of pizza drowned in four different cheeses.

In other contexts, psychologists have referred to this as the 'hedonic treadmill', which is a great metaphor likening the experience to one where we're constantly running, as though on a treadmill, chasing that carrot and never actually getting anywhere! As a result, we don't ever really get to experience as much joy or satisfaction as we'd like. And in fact we're often just left feeling frustrated, disappointed and downright miserable.

Of course there is no other aspect of our lives where the 'hedonic treadmill' is more evident than in our modern-day eating behaviours. We can supersize our movie meals for just 50 cents more. McDonald's (and its 'golden arches' branding) is now officially more widely recognised as a cultural icon than the Christian cross. These days, we're served up pasta on gigantic plates—enough not only to give us the Dolmio grin, but the double (and triple) chins to go with it. And compared to the standard family-sized bottle of soft drink of the 1960s, which was a mere 750 millilitres, we're now looking at super-duper three-litre ones. And we're still not satisfied!

To combat this growing problem, most popular diet interventions include a lot of pill-popping, restrictive eating, punishing exercise routines and negativity; they're often punitive and even insulting approaches to weight loss. In effect, they play right into the hands of the 'tyranny of when' by encouraging dieters to think they'll be happy when they've lost a certain number of kilograms or dropped however many dress sizes. Accordingly, many people feel depressed, hopeless and helpless when they're blamed for being overweight or labelled as lazy, ill-disciplined failures.

So why is my approach, The Happiness Diet, any different? Thanks for asking. I'll tell you why.

Whereas most diets propose that if you lose weight then you'll be happy, The Happiness Diet proposes that if you get happy first then you'll lose weight!

And the good news is that this isn't something I just made up. Rather, it's based on a growing groundswell of scientific literature that supports the 'positivity' approach to weight loss—as well as to many other areas of life.

Traditionally, psychologists have focused on negative emotions and as a result we know quite a bit about how they affect us.

wellbeing. Without adequate sleep, we simply won't enjoy a happy and healthy life (at any age!).

2. Make sleep a priority—too often sleep is seen as a waste of time or not as important as other health behaviours such as exercise. But it is just as important, and if it's not seen as a priority and is sacrificed for other things, then that will have a detrimental effect on your health.

3. Eat well (as described earlier)—but avoid eating too much, especially late at night. Also avoid excessive consumption of caffeine (especially in the late afternoon or evening) and alcohol.

4. Keep active—the benefits of activity and exercise were described earlier in terms of physical health and psychological wellbeing, but exercise during the day also improves the quality and quantity of sleep at night.

5. Learn to relax—as already noted, worry and stress are some of the most common causes of insomnia and of sleep difficulties but simple and applied relaxation strategies are very effective in helping people get to sleep initially and get back to sleep if they wake during the night.

6. Develop a good sleep routine—we are, mostly, creatures of habit and having good sleep habits can make an enormous difference to our ability to sleep well. So try to ensure you go to bed at the same time every night and that you get up at the same time every morning (even if you've not slept all that well).

7. Manage your time well during the day—this helps minimise stress, which, as flagged above, can often impair sleep. Work out and focus on what's most important and try not to get

distracted by seemingly (but not really) urgent issues or by useless, non-productive or non-pleasurable activities.

8. Develop healthy thinking—do this to avoid worry and to increase feelings of hope and optimism. People tend to sleep much better when they feel good about their lives and when they're looking forward to the future (this will be described in much more detail in the next chapter, Chapter Four).

9. Address other problems—worries, whether they be physical, psychological, financial or to do with relationships, if left unresolved will contribute to ongoing stress and this, as we know, is not healthy. So take action and/or seek help from a friend, family member or even a professional.

10. Practise and persevere—like most things, change can take time and be hard work. If you've not been sleeping well in the past it could take a while before you experience improvements. But for most people the strategies in this list will be very likely to work; as long as you stick at them and persevere for at least a few weeks. If you're still struggling after that then, as in any other area, it might be wise to have a full assessment with an appropriate health professional.

This component of health and wellbeing doesn't end with sleep; it's also important to ensure you get adequate rest to allow your body and your mind to recover and recuperate from day-to-day stress and pressures.

Although meditation and relaxation have been dismissed in the past as 'fringe' behaviours, they have become increasingly mainstream and this is largely because there is so much evidence proving their many and varied benefits. Regardless of age, mindfulness and meditation can, for example:

- reduce stress and depression;
- improve cognitive functioning (thinking, memory and decision-making);
- help manage pain;
- protect the brain against mental illness and some forms of age-related decline;
- improve self-awareness and emotional regulation;
- enhance compassion (for oneself and for others);
- decrease your chances of getting sick and improve your chances of recovering more quickly if you do get sick;
- improve sleep.

As if all these benefits were not enough, a team of researchers from the University of California, Los Angeles, found that meditating for half an hour every day could help older people feel less lonely. Learning to focus on the present instead of dwelling on the past or worrying about the future can stop people from feeling alone and unloved, the study concluded.

This is particularly important because as people age, partners and spouses are more likely to die and children increasingly scatter and/or become busier, making them less able to spend time with their parents. Loneliness can then set in, which, other studies have found, is associated with the increased risk of heart disease, Alzheimer's disease, depression and even premature death. In fact experts warn that being lonely can be just as bad for health as smoking and obesity! (Which is why I will address comprehensively the development and maintenance of positive relationships in Chapter Six.)

If you've never meditated before, here are some simple suggestions to get you started:

- Begin by setting aside some time, each and every day, when you won't be disturbed (and if you're a newcomer to meditation I'd strongly encourage you to commit to 2–4 weeks of regular practice, at the very least, to ensure you give it a fair trial before determining its success or otherwise).
- Find a quiet place where you can sit (or lie) comfortably and ideally return to the same place each and every day.
- Make yourself comfortable and take a few, slow breaths.
- Don't necessarily try to change anything or even to achieve anything; just practise for the sake of practice and know that you'll be doing yourself some good.
- Now begin by taking a few deep, slow breaths (just two or three) and then allow your breathing to settle into its own natural rhythm; don't force it at all.
- As your breathing becomes comfortable and relaxed, begin to focus your mind on it; you'll notice that your chest and stomach rise slightly as you breathe in, and then lower slightly as you breathe out.
- Continue to focus on this feeling of the air passing in and out through your nose and/or mouth and begin to repeat the following two words, quietly and gently: 'in' as you breathe in and, 'relax' as you breathe out.
- Continue this for as long as you can; as you do so, you'll notice that from time to time your mind will wander.

- Reassure yourself that this is perfectly normal and quite OK. All you need to do, as soon as you become aware of your wandering mind, is gently ease it back to focusing on your breathing, and those two simple words—'in' and 'relax'.

And that's all there is to it! It's pretty simple, really, although as you'll find as soon as you start to practise, simple is not always easy.

The biggest problem most people experience with meditation is frustration and/or disappointment when they find their mind wandering and/or when they notice they're being distracted by other thoughts, sounds or sensations in their body. But that frustration mostly comes from unrealistic expectations such as 'I should be able to focus for longer' or 'I should be able to clear or empty my mind'.

Both of those expectations are unrealistic and unhelpful because it's not possible to 'empty' or completely 'clear' one's mind. What is possible, however, is the ability to focus on one thing only (such as those two words or a mantra or a prayer), but like most things, this takes practice and for the majority of us, we'll probably only ever get to the point where we can maintain our focus for a few minutes at a time. Maintaining focus for that amount of time, though, is absolutely fine; as long as we refocus as often and as quickly as we can and as long as we practise several times a day. There's no need to spend hours on this (unless you want to!) but if you can set aside 3–5 minutes, 3–5 times each day (and then build from there when you're ready) you'll be doing extremely well and you'll start to enjoy the many wonderful benefits that come from the regular practice of relaxation- and meditation strategies.

In the broader discussion on meditation, a specific type of meditation that focuses on compassion has been shown to also improve immune-system function; that is, it actually helps the body's natural healing systems.

In a meditation centre high up in the mountains of Colorado, visitors spend up to ten hours each day, for up to two or three months, sitting in silence, hoping to experience what might be called 'enlightenment'. This style of meditation, modelled on the lifestyles of Indian and Japanese monks, helps many westerners in their search for better health, wellbeing and happiness.

Interestingly, in 2007, the retreat allowed a group of scientists to stay to try to answer the very simple question of whether the meditation practices were 'doing any good'. So as the visitors contemplated and reflected upon love and compassion, joy and happiness, the researchers measured brainwave activity, heart rates and a multitude of other physical and behavioural variables.

Many of the findings were quite expected, as much research had previously been conducted into the positive effects and benefits of meditation. Improvements were found, for example, in cognitive functioning and wellbeing. But one finding was considered to be quite surprising and, in fact, extremely exciting. Meditation, it was discovered, protected the 'caps' on the ends of the chromosomes (those telomeres I referred to in Chapter One) and as a result, stopped the ends from fraying. What this meant, in simple terms, was that meditation, via its impact on telomeres, could potentially delay the process of ageing. When I first read that I thought to myself, *Wow!*

There are many types of meditation but one of the most prac-tised, and most researched, is mindfulness meditation, which 'pathways of restoration and enhancement', possibly improving the functioning of the parasympathetic nervous system or causing the production of growth hormone.

Whatever the reasons for these amazingly positive and powerful benefits, for those who'd like to live a longer and better, healthier and happier life I'd suggest they start meditating now!

IN BETWEEN CHAPTERS THREE AND CHAPTER FOUR

I THOUGHT IT WOULD BE HELPFUL TO . . .

. . . comment briefly on the interconnectedness of our bodies and minds. I'm not referring, here, to anything esoteric or 'alternative' but rather to a universal reality: that our psychological- and biological makeup are closely integrated.

This is in direct contrast to Cartesian dualism (the belief that mind and matter are two independent entities), which is a very outdated concept and one that has little place in modern thinking—especially when it comes to health and wellbeing. Consider, for example, the following:

- Exercise is obviously good for our physical fitness and strength but it's also one of the most effective stress-management tools and antidepressants so it's also very good for our mental health and psychological wellbeing.
- Anxiety and stress are emotions and therefore psychological but anyone that's experienced either knows that they have a

significant physical effect (e.g. muscle tension, increased heart rate, sweating).

So if we're to take a comprehensive approach to health and well-being we need to address the physical and the psychological. Chapter Three covered the main aspects of physical health so now it's time to move on to Chapter Four and a discussion about some of the 'big guns' of psychological health.

CHAPTER 4

COPING STYLES, MENTAL HEALTH AND HAPPINESS (HOPE, OPTIMISM AND PLAY)

'When I was five years old, my mother always told me that happiness was the key to life. When I went to school, they asked me what I wanted to be when I grew up. I wrote down "happy". They told me I didn't understand the assignment, and I told them they didn't understand life.'
JOHN LENNON

One of the inspirations for writing this book came from some research I stumbled upon a few years ago, referring to the potential benefits of medicines based on the active ingredient in red wine. The drugs are synthetic versions of resveratrol, which is found in the skin and seeds of grapes and is an organic chemical long thought to have a beneficial effect on health. In fact some claim that resveratrol and the artificial versions of it are believed to have an anti-ageing effect that ultimately has the potential to help people live until they're 150!

However, as with any drug intervention, its use causes unwanted side effects and bringing a safe version to the market will typically take much longer than many of us (and especially many journalists) hope. So in the meantime we'll have to settle for drinking red wine, in moderation, or engaging in other healthy behaviours that we know provide benefits now.

Amazingly, one of the simplest but most effective strategies we can use to promote health and wellbeing generally, and specifically in an ageing population, is adopting an attitude of optimism, happiness and positivity.

It's long been claimed that 'laughter is the best medicine' but rather than just being a saying, now we have real science to support this. An investigation involving a collaboration between the Arts Health Institute, the Humour Foundation, the University of New South Wales and the Dementia Collaborative Research group has been assessing, for a few years now, the possible impact of a weekly dose of smiles and laughs.

The Sydney Multisite Intervention of LaughterBosses and ElderClowns study (note the great acronym: SMILE) provides a daily regimen of jokes and silliness and, remarkably, it's replacing psychotropic and antidepressant drug use in dementia patients.

An August 2013 article on the project, published in the *Sydney Morning Herald*, quoted Barry Cowling, operations manager of Summit Care nursing home in Randwick (New South Wales), as saying that humour therapy had reduced aggression and depression among residents in the secure dementia wing of his facility.

'We've had residents where we could reduce psychotropic drugs or have them come off, and we could see benefits to staff with improvements in morale and engagement.'

And it happens that I know one of the people who were instrumental in the development and in the delivery of the intervention that was at the heart of this study.

About five or six years ago, a friend and colleague, Professor Marc Cohen (a world leader in wellness research and practice), invited me to speak at a health and wellness festival (Radiance) within a music festival (the Woodford Folk Festival in Queensland). This began a multi-year adventure for my family and I (combining me presenting and all of us having a great holiday) and also led to me meeting a wonderful man by the name of Jean-Paul Bell.

At Woodford, the first year we attended, Jean-Paul was helping out some friends at the Children's Festival, a self-contained area within the wider festival grounds, filled with fun activities and entertainment for younger people. As our children were quite young at the time my wife and I spent many hours there and I still remember, very fondly, watching my son learn basic magic and clowning tricks from this beautiful, humble and very talented man.

I subsequently discovered that Jean-Paul was much more than just a children's entertainer. He was a children's entertainer but he was also a 'legend' in the Australian entertainment industry, having been at the forefront of circus, clowning and vaudeville performance for several decades.

Just as impressive was the fact that I learned he was one of the founding fathers of the fantastic Clown Doctors (a program run by the Humour Foundation). As described on their website:

Clown Doctors dose sick children in hospital with fun and laughter!

Imagine being a child in hospital, away from the comfort of your home and all that is familiar, and feeling sad, anxious, frightened, lonely or in pain. This is where Clown Doctors can help. They treat children in hospital with medicine of a different kind . . . doses of fun and laughter!

Many kids in hospital face a hard time. Clown Doctors address the psychosocial needs of the child in hospital in a unique way. By parodying the hospital routine, the Clown Doctors help children feel less traumatised by medical procedures. Oversized medical equipment, 'red-nose' transplants, 'cat' scans, humour checks and funny bone examinations are all part of the fun. By exaggerating intimidating jargon and procedures, fear and anxiety are reduced.

'Clown Rounds' are conducted through all wards including intensive care and oncology, and most clinics including emergency and burns. Children can forget their illness for a moment and return to a world of fantasy and play. It is hard to keep a sad face when the Clown Doctors come in! It is not only laughter that is important. A smile, or a glimmer in the eye, is also a special moment.

Along with several other equally inspiring and dedicated people Jean-Paul set up the Clown Doctors in 1996 and performed the role (excuse the pun!) of Creative Director for just over twenty years. For a variety of personal and professional reasons he left the Humour Foundation a few years ago but he continued doing work that was just as important, shifting his focus from children to elders and from laughter to play!

In 2011, Jean-Paul brought together another impressive group of people (including his highly qualified wife) and established what's now known as the Arts Health Institute. It's a not-for-profit

organisation whose mission is to integrate, through research, education and the delivery of programs, creative arts into health care.

As described in their promotional material:

> The Arts Health Institute believes that the arts enrich our lives
> and when we are ill or infirm we need creative engagement
> more than ever. We bring creativity to care by playfully inte-
> grating the Arts into the health and aged care communities to
> enable life changing programs in hospitals, aged care facilities
> and in the general community. AHI provides education for
> professional artists and health workers and programs that are
> designed to foster positive interaction between staff and clients
> and their families.

When I interviewed Jean-Paul for this book he made a comment
that struck me to the core; he said, quite matter-of-factly when
I think back on it, that a lack of play is similar to a lack of
sleep—they are both forms of deprivation. Another interviewee,
Maggie Beer (to whom I'll refer in more detail in Chapter 8),
made a very similar point about quality food in aged care. As a
well-known Australian cook and food author, she's obviously very
passionate about quality food but more than just being important
for nutrition and health, Maggie sees quality food as being integral
to quality of life (but more on that later).

Returning to Jean-Paul and the Arts Health Institute, rather
than clowning (which Jean-Paul determined to be not completely
appropriate for an aged population), their core program is now
based on a valet-type character, like the sort you'd see out the
front of or in the elevator of an old-style hotel (think back to

the early twentieth century). And as already noted, the focus is not just on laughter and humour (although my observations of Jean-Paul and his programs have involved much of both) but more generally, play.

Jean-Paul's work in this area has been greatly influenced by the internationally renowned Dr Stuart Brown, founder of the National Institute for Play, based in California.

Much of Dr Brown's work has focused on play amongst children but he and many others believe play is just as important for adults, and especially for older adults. Around the time I was researching this section of the book (and just after I spoke at the Arts Health Institute's National 'Play up!' conference) I posted a tweet (a 140-character-or-fewer comment on Twitter) inviting anyone and everyone to 'play for more happiness'.

My son happened to see it and commented that it was cool but then paused, thought, and commented again in a questioning tone, 'But grown-ups don't play, do they?'

Unfortunately, his belief is all too common and we all lose out as a result. Just as sadly, play is all too often equated with silliness—being unproductive, involving useless frivolity and, among other things, a lack of responsibility. Accordingly, whenever the idea of play is brought up in the context of anyone over the age of eighteen (or even twelve), it's considered inappropriate, irrelevant and even downright dangerous.

For most people, the belief is that once they've put on the suit and tie, literally and metaphorically, life is way too serious for play and play is so far down the list of priorities that it becomes, effectively, unimportant.

But why is this the case? And is it helpful or useful?

Well, I'm not 100 per cent sure about the answer to the first question but I am pretty sure about the answer to the second one; and in my humble opinion the answer is a resounding 'No.'

Play creates positive emotion and positive emotion produces numerous benefits (including improved health and wellbeing, innovation and creativity, collaboration and a better ability to relate to and with others). Play is also stimulating and energising and which adults don't want or need more stimulation and/or energy?

Having spent several decades reviewing the role of play in a range of different contexts, Dr Stuart Brown believes that play exists naturally all around us, all the time, but we typically only notice it when it's absent. And when it's absent it can contribute to a number of significant problems.

He's found that lack of play can predict criminal behaviour; and that the appropriate use of play can markedly and positively enhance satisfaction within relationships. In their book *The Levity Effect*, Adrian Gostick and Scott Christopher also cite numerous studies proving that it even 'pays to lighten up' in the workplace.

Research from the Great Place to Work Institute's database (which includes more than one million people), for example, reveals that 'great' companies consistently score higher marks for 'fun' than their less-great peers. (More than 80 per cent of employees within the 'great' companies reported feeling as though they were working in a 'fun environment'.) The research is pretty clear—the best companies are having the best time.

And the best managers also seem to get and keep the best employees (which might go at least part of the way to explaining the aforementioned findings). The international research firm, Ipsos, conducted a study in 2006 exploring the relationship between a manager's sense of humour (as rated by his or her employees) and employee retention (how likely the employees were to say that they'd still be in their current job, one year on). Once again, the results were pretty clear-cut—employees who rated their manager's sense of humour as 'above average' rated the likelihood that they'd still be in their job twelve months on at almost 90 per cent; but employees who rated their manager's sense of humour as 'average' or as 'below average' rated their changes of staying on at only 77 per cent.

Taking a different, but equally important, perspective humour and play have been shown to provide many physical and psychological benefits. Stress can reduce blood flow whereas play and laughter can increase blood flow (which can provide the same benefits as exercise!). Even anticipating something funny can have benefits including, according to research conducted by Dr Lee Berk, Assistant Professor of Family Medicine at the University of Maryland, reducing levels of at least four of the neuroendocrine hormones associated with stress. Looking forward to and enjoying play can reduce stress and depression, as well as anger, tension and fatigue.

Taking all of this into account, Gostick and Christopher conclude, 'for this reason, Hal Rosenbluth, CEO of Rosenbluth International, the nation's largest travel services company with $2 billion in revenues, considers it "almost inhumane if companies create a climate where people can't naturally have fun". From his perspective, "our role and responsibility as leaders and associates is to create a place where people can enjoy themselves. I know our company is doing great when I walk around and hear people laughing. The enjoyment translates into performance."'

And is there any reason why this theory should not apply in other contexts, whether at a place of business, home, aged-care facility or indeed anywhere else? I certainly can't think of one!

•

Although the results of the SMILE study are impressive, most involved in this type of work agree that it's not just the laughter and the humour that works the magic (although this helps), but just as importantly the benefits can probably be attributed to engaging with and connecting to the patients, giving them a sense of hope that things can get better. Too many dementia patients and too many who treat them (or family members who support them) suffer from a sense of therapeutic nihilism—that there's nothing that works or that will help!

One of the things that struck me when I interviewed Frank (the runner) and Petrea (the inspirational helper about whom I'll write much more in Chapter Nine)—and, in fact, all of the wonderful people who were generous enough to talk with me about their lives and loves and thoughts on ageing—was the energy they had for life and the hope they had for the future. Accordingly, they didn't just continue to live full and active lives but they also continued to plan for full and active futures.

A great example of this was Paul Clitheroe, one of Australia's best-known and most-respected commentators on finances and money, who was one of the first people who agreed to being interviewed but who also told me that it would have to wait a few weeks because he was just about to head overseas to climb Mount Kilimanjaro! He was just about to turn 60 years of age.

Ageing well, I've come to learn, involves not just having an attitude that holds few limits (as we saw from Ellen Langer's amazing research) but also from adopting an attitude that the future is bright. All of those I interviewed and about whom I read mentioned something along the lines of believing—and I mean really believing—that they still had plenty of living to do and even, in many cases, that their best years were ahead of them.

This shouldn't really be a huge surprise because several decades of psychological research have shown, quite clearly, that hope and optimism are key contributors to happiness, health and success.

In fact, if you control all other variables, research shows that optimists will live longer than pessimists. They also get sick less often and if they do get sick they recover more quickly. In addition, they perform better in almost every area of life and they have better-quality relationships (which also make a significant positive contribution to health and happiness).

I grew up with a pretty amazing example of living, breathing optimism. My great-aunt Lilly was always one of the favourites at family gatherings simply because she never complained, continuously smiled, and always had a good word to say about others, her life and the world.

And it's not as though she had it easy.

In fact Aunty Lilly (the fact we called her 'Aunty' instead of 'Great Aunty' was indicative of her youthful and positive attitude to life) had it pretty tough. Her husband lost his eyesight relatively young and so couldn't work, which meant Lilly was the primary carer and breadwinner. As she aged she also began to experience a range of her own significant vision-related and other physical health problems.

And this is just the short version of her long and at times quite complex story, but I can't recall ever hearing her complain; not even once. And I only remember the staff in the nursing home where she eventually was forced to move, talking about her in resoundingly positive terms.

In fact I asked her once how she stayed so positive despite a growing list of challenges and limitations. Her response could have come straight from the handbook of optimism:

'What's the point of complaining?' she said. 'I'm still alive; I can still talk to my friends and sit outside and enjoy the sun and . . .' And she went on to recite a long list of relatively simple tasks and activities that most of us would take for granted. It's this attitude of focusing more on what she had and less on what she didn't have that I believe helped her to continue living a happy life.

This approach brings to mind the 'first cousin' of optimism and positivity, which is gratitude. If you remember back to the Blue Zone communities, gratitude was one of the common features that threaded its way through the fabric of life in Sardinia and Okinawa and the other remarkable towns and cities mentioned.

Not all that surprisingly, gratitude and appreciation have been widely studied and their benefits repeatedly acknowledged. Professor Robert Emmons of the University of California has largely led the way in gratitude research and his list of publications (academic articles and books) would fill a whole chapter. But his work, and that of many others, can be summed up pretty simply: gratitude works; gratitude pays; if you practise appreciation on a regular basis you will live better and longer.

This is not necessarily a new idea as the notion of 'giving thanks' dates back to the fundamentals of every major religion and school of philosophical thought. But what is new and what we have available now that we didn't necessarily have ten, twenty or 30 years ago is, firstly: strong evidence to support the idea that gratitude is good for our psychological and physical health and wellbeing and, secondly: proven and practical strategies we can recommend and teach people, knowing, with a great deal of confidence, that if and when utilised and applied will lead to significant benefits.

You might be wondering, then, what these 'proven and practical' gratitude strategies are.

Well, I'm glad you asked and I'm very happy to provide you with some of my favourites:

- Three Good Things—at the end of each day, write down three good things that have occurred in the last 24 hours.
- What Went Well (WWW)—similar to the Three Good Things exercise, WWW invites you to focus on those things in your day that have been positive, led to successful outcomes or anything that happened from which you've enjoyed some sort of positive process.
- Gratitude Journals—regularly writing down all the best things in your life, all those things for which you're grateful and appreciative, has also been found to be extremely useful. You can even include unpleasant or negative life events if in some way or other you're grateful for the lesson(s) learned. This is similar to the previous two strategies described but is more general, not limited to any specific number of things or the last 24 hours and typically involves a greater depth of emotionality and writing than the more simple list-making.

- A fourth and final proven favourite is to write a gratitude letter and make a gratitude visit. The simplest version of this (although like any other recommendation in this book, you're more than welcome to modify or adapt it to suit your personality and/or circumstances) involves taking the following steps:
  - think about someone in your life who's had a positive influence;
  - call that person and organise to meet within the next few weeks;
  - in the intervening period of time, write them a (short) letter outlining what they did and why you're grateful;
  - go to the meeting, engage in the usual greetings and small talk, then, at an appropriate time, read them the letter (you can even give them the letter as a tangible reminder of the experience).

Typically, the gratitude visit is a profoundly positive experience, for both people, which is why it is such an important exercise. Although all forms of appreciation are beneficial, most are helpful only for you, the individual practising. But the gratitude visit incorporates another essential aspect of this significant emotion: as well as *experiencing* gratitude it's also important to *express* it. That way, the positive emotion and other gains are multiplied and spread even more widely, which is a great outcome for all involved.

Unfortunately Aunty Lilly didn't live to read this book but she did live to the ripe old age of 98 and was still smiling (pretty much most of the time) up until her dying day.

And Aunty Lilly's example to us is consistent with the findings of a fascinating study conducted by Sarah Pressman (from the cereals, wholemeal bread, fruit, dried fruit, dried peas, beans and lentils, all of which are excellent sources of fibre.

- In short, the more 'natural' foods you eat and the less 'processed' and 'packaged' foods the better.

Although these are the general recommendations, it may also be worthwhile consulting your local general practitioner or, better still, a qualified dietician or nutritionist if you're in any way unsure about what or how much to eat for optimum health and wellbeing.

It's also important to offer a note of caution when modifying your dietary habits. There are many who'll claim that a particular diet or meal plan will provide the secret to healthy living and to positive ageing; some go so far as to argue certain foodstuffs will prevent ageing and keep you younger. The evidence supporting these claims, however, is not all that strong.

I don't think any of us really know as much as we'd like to when it comes to providing specific dietary or nutritional advice for living well or for ageing well, but something we can all do—and indeed I would encourage you to do—is follow the evidence-based recommendations listed above and the current dietary guidelines as well as avoid those things that have been proven to contribute to poor health or even to early mortality. (There's little argument about the powerful association between cigarette- and alcohol abuse earlier in life and health and wellbeing later in life, for example.) So, eat as healthily as you can but avoid at all costs excessive consumption of alcohol (although drinking in moderation is fine) and the smoking of cigarettes.

While it is important to be conscious of what and how much we eat, something else to keep in mind is how we eat and with whom.

As referred to earlier, Epicurus had some wise words to say about eating and in addition to noting that we should be happy with less he also recommended, 'one should never eat alone' and that 'the pleasures of the table [include] . . . those of conversation.'

Just as dance has proven to be a fantastic form of exercise due to its combination of physical exertion, mental effort and social interaction, so too can eating provide a healthy way in which to socialise. It's in our interests, especially from a psychological point of view, to ensure that all aspects of life are as enjoyable as possible. So if eating well can be combined with positive social interaction, then we create a double win.

While other apparently contradictory research points to the benefits of eating without distraction, these findings—and their associated recommendations—need not necessarily be mutually exclusive.

Mindful eating has increasingly been recommended in recent years as a vital cog in the wheel of healthy eating and, for many, in successful weight loss. Mindfulness can be defined as 'observing without judgement and with curiosity' and mindful eating, therefore, can be considered as the art of being aware of the food we consume and of the process of consumption.

A number of studies have shown that mindful eating is correlated with eating less and enjoying the eating more (yet another double win!). The concept of mindful eating is a part of a psychological weight-management program I developed at The Happiness Institute several years ago. The Happiness Diet recognises that weight management (and in some cases weight loss) is not just a diet- and activity-related issue (what and how much we eat, as well as how much we move and exercise), but is also

University of Kansas) and colleagues. The authors studied the autobiographies of a number of professionals looking for words and phrases that were high in (or representative of) positive emotion and those that were high in (or representative of) negative emotion. They then correlated these findings with longevity.

What they found provided more strong evidence for the benefits of happiness and feeling good. In their conclusion they stated:

> After controlling for sex, year of publication, health (based on disclosed illness in autobiography), native language, and year of birth, the use of more activated positive emotional words (e.g., lively, vigorous, attentive, humorous) was associated with increased longevity.

So people who described their own lives, in their own writings, in more positive ways, actually lived longer!

And before we move on it's worth noting that we're not just talking about living a few extra days, weeks or even months here. Rather, those whose words were assessed to include significantly more positive emotion lived up to six years longer than those using more negative expressions.

And if you want more evidence to support the rationale for optimistic thinking then you might also be interested in a wonderful study from the Netherlands, published in the American psychiatry journal, *JAMA*.

The authors of this study begin by reminding us of the fact that depression can kill. That is, a significant number of studies have shown that major depression is associated with higher rates of cardiovascular morbidity. But the authors of this study wanted to see if the opposite was true: if pessimism and depression can shorten life, can optimism and happiness lengthen life?

Well, the answer is a pretty resounding yes.

Just under 1000 men and women, aged between 65 and 85, were asked by the researchers to complete a range of health and wellbeing questionnaires, including one that measured optimism. All of the subjects were then followed up over the next nine or so years. During this period of time there were 397 deaths. What's interesting, however, is what one finds when one compares the most optimistic with the most pessimistic in this sample.

Beginning by looking at the information for all those who had died, the data analysis found that the pessimists were twice as likely to die as the optimists. If one then looked specifically at cardiovascular-related deaths, the pessimists were four times more likely to die.

Not surprisingly, then, the authors concluded that their findings supported the notion that optimism protects against death; it helps people live longer and healthier. And the good news is we can all learn to be more optimistic!

Joseph Conrad, author of *Heart of Darkness*, the famous novel behind the arguably even more famous movie, *Apocalypse Now*, once cautioned, 'woe to the man whose heart has not learned while young to hope, to love, to put its trust in life', as though if these lessons are not learned early on then there is no hope.

Thankfully, Conrad was not correct—either in my humble opinion or in those expressed by the published research in this area. Martin Seligman, for example, one of the most influential and highly regarded psychologists of the modern era, coined the phrase 'learned optimism'. In stark contrast to Conrad's bleak

In short, when we experience negative emotions (such as fear or anxiety) we close up; we tend to withdraw physically and psychologically and as a result we tend not to cope with our problems as well.

In contrast, the more modern psychological science of positivity shows that positive emotions lead to improved performance, coping and resilience via the broadening of our minds and the increased capacity to build on previous experiences.

What this means for your weight management is that positive emotions are not just 'nice', they're also much, much more than that. In fact, they're downright powerful and will turbo-charge your chances of success. How? Because when you experience appropriate positive emotions you become significantly more motivated, energised and inspired to do what you need to do to achieve your goals and so you markedly boost your chances of success by putting positivity first and foremost.

What this all means is that now, rather than succumbing to the *tyranny* of when, you can harness the *power* of then. By this I mean that you can use the idea of creating happiness first in order to *then* achieve more of your goals.

How great would that be? You get to enjoy the wonders of positive emotions both before and after succeeding in your efforts.

So by all means address, as noted above, the content of your diet and especially the sizes of your portions, but please don't ignore the psychological aspects of eating and weight management as for many people these are just as (if not more) important contributors to the ultimate goal of achieving and maintaining a healthy weight.

Sleep and rest

Finally, it's important to stress what could be considered obvious: that it's hard to be happy if you're tired all the time. And unfortunately many of us *are* tired much of the time.

Although some of this can be attributed to issues raised in the previous sections (reduced or inadequate activity levels can compromise good quality and an adequate quantity of sleep, for example) and the fact that the sleep requirements of the average person actually decline slightly with age so we need a bit less anyway, research still suggests that the average Australian gets at least one hour's less sleep each night than he or she needs and, sadly, sleep problems tend to be more prevalent in the elderly.

In addition to a general feeling of tiredness, however, there is a range of health and medical problems that become more common with age and that directly or indirectly impact upon sleep. These include Alzheimer's disease, chronic pain (including arthritis), cardiovascular disease, neurological conditions and bladder or urinary problems. But for many, the cause of sleep difficulties will be insomnia and the cause of this, in most cases, is worry or stress.

The good news is that the majority of sufferers can take a few relatively simple steps to improve their sleep. I wrote about this in my very first book, *The Good Sleep Guide: Ten Steps to Better Sleep and How to Break the Worry Cycle*, which included the following ten practical tips for better sleeping:

1. Understand the need for sleep—sleep is a vitally important biological function, needed for our physical and psychological

pessimism, Seligman confidently argued that although there were undoubtedly some who were naturally optimistic, others could learn to be.

Seligman could state this confidently because he was aware of a plethora of research (much of which he had conducted himself) supporting the notion. Optimism can be viewed as a skill and just like any other skill it can be taught and learned, practised and refined. In improving their abilities in this very helpful thinking style, people can increasingly enjoy its numerous resultant benefits.

Cognitive Therapy, Cognitive Behaviour Therapy and, more recently, Mindfulness Based (or Mindfulness Integrated) Cognitive Therapy and a range of similar approaches applied to myriad psychological issues (from depression to anxiety, drug- and alcohol abuse to weight management and eating disorders, and even to the improving of job satisfaction, employee wellbeing and productivity in the workplace) have achieved remarkable results by, in simple terms, helping people change the way they think about the world around them, the people with whom they interact and, sometimes most importantly of all, the way they think about themselves.

In short, contemporary psychology has largely been based on the well-supported premise that what happens to you is not quite as important as how you think about what happens to you; and there are always multiple ways to think about what's happening to you so the skill is in learning how to choose the most helpful interpretations. This is what optimism effectively is (although it's often referred to in the research by a number of other names, such as attributional or explanatory style).

Let me give you a specific example. Mary's shopping in her usual grocery store when she sees her neighbour, Susan. She politely waves but Susan wanders past without returning the greeting.

Oh dear, she thinks. *What have I done to upset her? I'm always upsetting people; she'll never forgive me or speak to me again!*

Not surprisingly, Mary was quite upset. If we look closely at Mary's interpretation of this seemingly innocuous interaction with Susan, we can see why: she followed all the rules of pessimism. Pessimists tend to view negative life events as being internal, general and permanent; that is, that everything is their fault and that it will always be bad. If you reflect on Mary's interpretation you'll notice that she blamed herself for everything and predicted it would always be terrible. Quite an overreaction one might assume.

But let's just imagine for a minute that Mary has magically been turned into an optimist. Now let's begin by noting that optimists are not Pollyanna, rose-coloured-glasses-type deniers. They do look for positives wherever and whenever possible but they also face up to cold hard realities (in a constructive way).

As an optimist, and an optimist who's grounded in reality, Mary (version two) might start by noting that the lack of response was a bit upsetting, but following this her interpretation would differ markedly from that of Mary (version one) and it might go something like this:

Oh, that's strange that Susan didn't acknowledge me. But maybe she was distracted or worried about something. Maybe I should call her later and check if everything is OK.

In stark contrast to the pessimistic internal, general and permanent interpretation of before, this second way was more external, specific and temporary; that is, Mary didn't assume it was all her fault, she certainly didn't generalise beyond this single incident to all other relationships and there was no hint that she was concerned that her friendship with Susan would be irreparably damaged.

As a result, Mary (version two) would be far less distressed by the incident and far more likely to behave in a constructive and helpful way afterwards.

Now here comes the crucial bit: we can all learn to think like Mary (version two)—we can all learn to think like optimists. I can state this confidently because I've read hundreds of scientific articles and books on the topic, I've seen it work with my clients and I've experienced change in myself.

But before going on to look at how, specifically, this can be achieved, it's worth noting this doesn't just apply to the treatment of psychological disorders or to the times we're required to cope with negative life events; optimism is also very relevant and important for dealing with positive life events.

Let's reacquaint ourselves with Mary. Instead of being ignored by her friend Susan (or thinking she's been ignored), this time Mary's just received some news from her husband, Barry. Barry has recently returned home and told her that she's been appointed to the board of a local club in which she's been very involved for many years. He is, understandably, very excited and pleased for her. Mary (version one) the pessimist is not, however, as excited. Her response to her husband Barry goes something like this: 'Oh dear, I'm not at all happy about this. They must have made a mistake appointing me; and even though this might seem good now, I'm sure it will be very stressful and there are already enough problems in my life right now! I just don't know how I'll cope!'

What's interesting about pessimists is that whereas they typically interpret negative life events as being internal (their fault), general (examples of how everything is bad) and permanent (never-ending), they change tack when faced with positive life events and see them as external (due to luck or error on someone's behalf), specific (not representative of how bad everything else in their life is) and temporary (good things never last).

So even when good things happen to pessimists like Mary they don't get to enjoy them!

But wait, we have (remember) two versions of Mary. There is, also, the optimistic Mary who when confronted by the same situation would respond quite differently and say something like this: 'Wow, this is fantastic! I've worked really hard for this [internal—taking credit for the achievement]; it's just an example of how great my life is at the moment [general] and it's going to be a fantastic few years with a great group of people [permanent—the good times will last].'

As hinted earlier, the really good news is that we can all learn to think like optimists—like Mary (version two). How do we do this? Well, quite simply, by following these four simple but powerful steps:

Four steps to thinking more optimistically

1. *Become more aware of your thinking*—most of us aren't even conscious of our thoughts and so the first step is to become more mindful of what's going through your mind. You can't change something if you don't even know what it is, so start thinking more about your thinking; write down your thoughts

and inner 'self-talk' at regular intervals and generally make a conscious effort to become more aware of what you say to yourself and how you interpret the events taking place in your day-to-day life.

2. *Remember that there are different ways of thinking about things*—as noted above (in the examples featuring Mary), there are always different ways of thinking about things. They are not necessarily 'right' or 'wrong' but they do all have pros and cons, which means that for different people in different contexts some ways of thinking are more helpful and constructive than others. You don't have to accept or believe the first thought that pops into your head.

3. *Practise questioning, challenging or debating with yourself*—one of the most important aspects of this approach is to remember that just because you think something doesn't mean it's true. Thoughts are not facts, so if one way of thinking is not helpful you don't have to accept it; you can, instead, question yourself the same way you might question someone else during a discussion by using one or more of the following strategies:

   a. Consider alternative perspectives. Ask yourself whether there might be different ways of looking at the situation you're currently in; try, also, to imagine what someone else might think if they were facing whatever it is you're currently facing.

   b. Gather evidence to assess the validity or reality of the thought. Remember, again, that thoughts are not facts so ask yourself whether there's evidence to support your current beliefs and, if not, what might be a more realistic and helpful way of viewing the circumstances.

   c. Keep things in perspective; consider asking yourself questions such as, 'Is it really that bad?' and 'Will it seem so bad in a day, week, month or year?'

   d. Avoid making unhelpful assumptions and especially avoid blaming yourself excessively for things that may well not have been entirely your fault.

4. *Generate a more helpful and realistic thought or attitude*— ultimately, if you can question your original thoughts and challenge any beliefs or assumptions that may not have been helpful or realistic, you'll be able to generate a way of thinking, in this specific situation, that will help you arrive at a better outcome—a solution or way of coping that's beneficial for you and all involved. Once you reach this, try repeating it to yourself in the back of your mind, until it becomes embedded and accepted.

Before concluding this section, it's very important to note that ageing well—and indeed living well—is not just about positive emotions and optimistic thinking. I hope I've made the point that both of these (positive emotions and optimism) are very important and very useful, but this does not mean healthy and happy people never experience so-called 'negative emotions' (such as sadness or grief, anger or anxiety, frustration or irritability) or various forms of distress.

I don't even like to refer to 'negative emotions' because it implies that such feelings are, in some way, bad for you, yet if we think about it, it is clear that they have an important role to play. Without fear and anxiety, for example, we wouldn't live very long as these 'negative emotions' protect us from dangerous

Buddhists claim alleviates suffering by enabling the meditator to be less caught up in everyday stress. Rigorous scientific studies have supported the benefits of mindfulness-based meditative approaches, finding that they lower blood pressure, improve healing for physical problems such as psoriasis and even boost immune responses in those receiving certain vaccines. As if such supporting evidence weren't enough, then short courses in mindfulness have also been found to be more effective than drug treatments in preventing relapse in patients with recurrent depression.

The specific implications that this form of meditation may have for ageing, however, came about largely due to the interest of a psychologist, Elissa Epel, from the University of California. Epel was especially interested in what (if anything) the Colorado meditation retreat was doing to the participants' chromosomes. And for any sceptical readers out there, Epel collaborated on this project with Elizabeth Blackburn, who was the joint winner of the 2009 Nobel physiology or medicine prize for her work on telomeres.

To quote from an article that referred to this research, published in *The Guardian*, 'they [Epel and Blackburn] found that at the end of the retreat, meditators had significantly higher telomerase activity than the control group, suggesting that their telomeres were better protected. The researchers are cautious, but say that in theory this might slow or even reverse cellular ageing. "If the increase in telomerase is sustained long enough," says Epel, "it's logical to infer that this group would develop more stable and possibly longer telomeres over time."'

All academics will be cautious, with good reason, about such findings, but it is still very positive and exciting to think that something like meditation, that's so affordable and so teachable (with no negative side effects, unlike many drug treatments), could so easily improve health and wellbeing in the elderly and could, very possibly, enhance longevity and even reverse a significant part of the process of ageing.

What's just as exciting is that this research isn't alone. Other studies have also confirmed the positive effects of meditation, especially in the context of ageing, with numerous investigations finding it has a protective effect against cognitive decline. To cite just one example, published in the American journal *Neurobiology of Aging*, thirteen regular meditation practitioners were compared with thirteen healthy 'matched' controls and assessed via, among other things, anatomical brain imagery.

Meditators, it was found, did not show the same age-related changes the non-meditators showed and the differences were greatest in parts of the brain responsible for attentional processing and control. Specifically, according to the researchers from the Department of Psychiatry and Behavioural Sciences at Emory University in Georgia, 'These findings suggest that the regular practice of meditation may have neuroprotective effects and reduce the cognitive decline associated with normal aging.'

There's little doubt, then, that meditation has positive and protective anti-ageing effects. There are some questions, however, about how this occurs. But most researchers, including those referred to in the previous few paragraphs, agree that there are at least two ways in which meditation is beneficial. Firstly, by producing a calming and relaxing response in the body it reduces and minimises the ongoing negative effects of chronic stress and anxiety. Secondly, according to Epel, meditation might also trigger situations and/or risky behaviours. Similarly, sadness and grief are necessary, contributing as they do to maturation and the development of wisdom.

One of the most famous theories within the field of positive psychology openly acknowledges the presence and utility of negative emotions. The research of Barbara Fredrickson (an American professor of psychology at the University of North Carolina) famously led to what's come to be known as the 'positivity ratio'—the ideal ratio of positive to negative emotions.

And the magic number? 3:1. The people who have been assessed as being the happiest—those who are thriving and flourishing—tend to experience positive and negative emotions in those proportions.

There are a couple of important lessons for us to learn from Fredrickson's positivity ratio. Firstly, it's not 1000 to one or even 100 to one—although the three-to-one ratio can increase, and more positive emotions might provide more benefits, it only applies up until a certain point, after which more (positive emotions) doesn't necessarily equate to better (feeling happier). Where that point lies varies from person to person and from context to context but it's probably somewhere around ten or twelve to one. After that, the benefits tail off—we can have too much of a good thing.

The second lesson to be learned is that the ratio is not three, four, ten or any other number to zero—even the happiest people experience negative emotions, because negative emotions are a normal part of life.

Some research suggests that one of the reasons older people might be happier (as referred to earlier) is because they manage more effectively these so-called 'negative emotions'. In the study cited earlier (see Chapter Three), older adults were less likely than younger adults to feel angry and anxious in their everyday lives or when they were asked to perform a stressful task.

In addition, older adults scored higher on a test designed to measure how well participants accept their negative emotions. The researchers call this trait 'acceptance' or a tendency to be in touch with rather than avoid negative emotions.

Further, in the famous and hugely influential Harvard Study of Adult Development, led by George Vaillant, one of the key differentiators of the 'happy-well' group when compared to the 'sad-sick' group was what they referred to as a 'mature psychological coping style' in everyday life.

This mature coping style involved the use of altruism and humour but is important to keep in mind in the context of negative emotions, too, because it highlights and reminds us that even the healthiest and happiest of older people experienced distress and faced difficult times—they just coped with them better.

Other coping strategies

Optimism is a fantastically useful 'tool' but there are many other ways healthy and happy people cope and, ultimately, thrive and flourish.

Managing negative feelings with emotional regulation strategies is important but so too are the relatively new approaches that have received increasing attention in the last decade, thanks largely to the Positive Psychology movement, relating to the recognition and utilisation of strengths.

As this is a relatively new construct within psychology (and even newer in terms of its understanding by the general public), let's start by explaining, just briefly, what 'strengths', in this context, are.

Back when I studied clinical psychology we didn't focus much at all on individuals' strengths; it was pretty much all about faults and weaknesses, limitations and where they were going wrong in life. This approach was not completely inappropriate because many of the people I saw (and continue to see) in my clinical psychology practice did have faults and were going wrong in life and they needed, in some way or other, to address these issues or else they'd continue to trip over the same problems time and time again.

However, these people (and in fact all of us), despite their faults and shortcomings, also have strengths and positive attributes, and continuing research is increasingly supporting the idea that although addressing our problems is important we can gain much more by also building upon our strengths.

Within the Positive Psychology movement strengths are those innate abilities that make us come alive when we utilise them; strengths are those attributes which when used help us realise our full potential; strengths are positive traits, values in action, positive dispositions that when used appropriately in context contribute to and build good character.

Thomas Jefferson was once quoted as saying that 'Happiness is the aim of life, but virtue is the foundation of happiness.'

It was a belief in this very concept that essentially led to the birth of a conference in 1999, under the watchful eye of Martin Seligman (grandfather of the Positive Psychology movement), with a focus on bringing together researchers and research programs that encouraged healthy development. One of several offshoots of this gathering was, about a year later, the establishment of the Values in Action (VIA) Institute, where Christopher Peterson gathered together and ultimately led a team of social scientists to define and determine key contributors to 'good character'. (If Seligman was the 'grandfather' of Positive Psychology then Peterson was the kindly, much-loved 'uncle'.)

When speaking to the admirable and wise people I interviewed for this book, they all—in various ways—described living a life beyond themselves as individuals and referred in some way or other to believing in the importance of 'doing the right thing'. (I'll discuss this in more detail in Chapter Eight, when I specifically write about purpose and meaning.)

A friend of mine, for example, who was happy to talk to me about this book but who asked to remain anonymous (something that's typical of his strengths of modesty and humility), 'retired' from his high-profile job in financial services with enough money to ensure that he'd never have to work again. That's not, however, what he chose to do.

Rather than just stepping back and enjoying a life of decadence or even quiet and relaxation (which he certainly could have afforded to do) he spoke to me about feeling both grateful for all he had and obliged to do something with the wealthy position he now found himself in. He had a nice house, kids at good schools and pretty much everything he wanted (although I'm always struck by how simply he seems to live for someone with his level of wealth). What he wanted to do was 'the right thing' and for him 'the right thing' was to give back to society in some way. This is 'character' and is a central pillar on which living a good life beyond the simple pleasures of happiness and positive emotion rests.

In short, then, when we utilise our strengths and when we live with character we enjoy all manner of benefits. According to just a few of the many research papers published in this area, people who use their strengths on a regular basis and, ideally, in new ways are (among other things) happier, less stressed, less likely to become depressed, enjoy higher levels of wellbeing, perform better at work and report having more meaning in their lives. A number of similar studies also report that people who use their strengths are more resilient and cope better, which ultimately leads to them not only enjoying the good times but also coping more effectively with the tough times.

So, how do you use your strengths more? The first step is to identify what they actually are. A good option for doing this is to complete the free survey that's available online at http://www.viacharacter.org.

A less formal but still worthwhile option is to review the following table in which the 24 strengths from the VIA model are listed and described:

The VIA Classification of Character Strengths

Wisdom & knowledge

Signature Strength	What it means	Tick your strengths
Curiosity, Interest in the world	You're open to new experiences and like to take a flexible approach to most things. You don't just tolerate ambiguity; you're intrigued by it. Your curiosity involves a wide-eyed approach to the world and a desire to actively engage in novelty.	

Signature Strength	What it means	Tick your strengths
Love of Learning	You love learning new things. You love being an expert and/or being in a position where your knowledge is valued by others.	
Judgement, Critical Thinking, Open-Mindedness	It's important to you to think things through and to examine issues from all angles. You don't quickly jump to conclusions but instead, carefully weigh up evidence to make decisions. If the facts suggest you've been wrong in the past, you'll easily change your mind.	
Ingenuity, Originality, Practical Intelligence	You excel in finding new and different ways to approach problems and/or to achieve your goals. You rarely settle for simply doing things the conventional way, more often looking to find better and more effective approaches.	
Social and Emotional Intelligence	You have a good understanding of yourself and of others. You are aware of your own moods and how to manage them. You're also very good at judging the moods of others and responding appropriately to their needs.	
Perspective	This strength is a form of wisdom. Others seek you out to draw on your ability to effectively solve problems and gain perspective. You have a way of looking at the world that makes sense and is helpful to yourself and to others.	

Courage

Signature Strength	What it means	Tick your strengths
Valour, Bravery	You're prepared to take on challenges and deal with difficult situations even if unpopular or dangerous. You have the courage to overcome fear as well as the ability to take a moral stance under stressful circumstances.	

Signature Strength	What it means	Tick your strengths
Perseverance, Diligence, Industry	You finish what you start. You're industrious and prepared to take on difficult projects (and you finish them). You do what you say and sometimes you even do more.	
Integrity, Honesty	You're honest, speaking the truth as well as living your life in a genuine and authentic way. You're down to earth and without pretence.	

Humanity & love

Signature Strength	What it means	Tick your strengths
Kindness, Generosity	You're kind and generous to others, and never too busy to do a favour. You gain pleasure and joy from doing good deeds for others. In fact, your actions are often guided by other people's best interests. At the core of this particular strength is an acknowledgment of the worth of others.	
Loving, Being Loved	You place a high value on close and intimate relationships with others. More than just loving and caring for others, they feel the same way about you and you allow yourself to be loved.	

Justice

Signature Strength	What it means	Tick your strengths
Citizenship, Loyalty, Teamwork	You're a great team player, excelling as a member of a group. You are loyal and dedicated to your colleagues, always contributing your share and working hard for the good and success of the group.	

Signature Strength	What it means	Tick your strengths
Fairness, Equity	You do not allow your own personal feelings to bias your decisions about other people. Instead, you give everyone a fair go and are guided by your larger principles of morality.	
Leadership	You're a good organiser and you're good at making sure things happen. You ensure work is completed by you and also maintain good relationships among group members.	

Temperance

Signature Strength	What it means	Tick your strengths
Self-Control	You can easily keep your desires, needs and impulses in check when necessary or appropriate. As well as knowing what's correct you're able to put this knowledge into action.	
Discretion, Caution, Prudence	You're a careful person. You look before you leap. You rarely, if ever, say or do things you later regret. You typically wait until all options have been fully considered before embarking on any course of action. You look ahead and deliberate carefully, making sure long-term success takes precedence over shorter-term goals.	
Modesty, Humility	You don't seek or want the spotlight. You're happy for your accomplishments to speak for themselves but you don't ever seek to be the centre of attention. You don't necessarily see yourself as being special and others often comment on, and respect your modesty.	

Transcendence

Signature Strength	What it means	Tick your strengths
Appreciation of beauty and excellence	You're one of those people who stops to smell the roses. You appreciate beauty, excellence and skill.	
Gratitude	You are highly aware of all the good things that happen to you and you never take them for granted. Further, you take time to express your thanks and you appreciate the goodness in others.	
Hope, Optimism	You expect the best for the future and you plan and work to achieve it. Your focus is on the future and on a positive future at that. You know that if you set goals and work hard good things will happen.	
Spirituality, Faith, Sense of purpose	You have strong and coherent beliefs about the higher purpose and meaning of the world. You're also aware of your position in this world and in the larger scheme of things. This awareness shapes your beliefs which shape your daily actions; this is a strong source of comfort to you.	
Forgiveness, Mercy	If you're wronged you can forgive. You allow people a second chance. You're guided more by mercy than revenge.	
Playfulness, Humour	You like to laugh and to make others laugh and smile. You enjoy and are good at play. You easily see the light side of life.	
Passion, Enthusiasm	You're energetic, spirited and passionate. You wake up and look forward to most days. You throw yourself, body and soul, in to all activities you undertake.	

You might also like to visit www.viacharacter.org for more information about the history and development of Character Strengths

I strongly encourage you to set aside some time to review the list and to consider what you believe your top three strengths might be. Ideally, talk to your partner or a good friend about this as well and see what they think. Ask yourself questions such as:

- What do I most love doing?
- What energises me?
- What makes me feel most alive?
- What do I most look forward to?
- When do I feel most 'me'?

Identifying your top strengths is the first step towards using them and using them is an important step towards coping well with life, in thriving and flourishing at all stages and in all contexts.

So how then, once you've identified your strengths, do you use them more effectively and more often? Simply make a point of thinking about all the tasks and projects on which you work, in all areas of your life, and think about how you can approach them from the perspective of your top strengths.

Now try to apply your strengths in different ways, each and every week. If, for example, one of your top strengths is a love of learning then set aside time every day, week and/or month to learn something new. (Learn a new word every day, read a new book or watch a new educational video every week, study a new course each month or year.)

If, on the other hand, one of your top strengths is creativity then make sure you have time in your busy schedule for creating; for drawing or painting or writing or playing music (whatever your favoured form of creative expression may be).

Here are a few more examples of strengths and their possible applications in daily life:

- appreciation of beauty—visit new galleries or museums;
- bravery or courage—talk to your local politician about something you consider to be an injustice;
- gratitude—regularly record all the best things in your life;
- ability to love—write a note to someone special and hide it in a place where they'll find it during the next few days;
- zest—do at least a few things each day because you want to rather than because you have to.

As with most if not all of the suggestions made in this book there are no answers that are perfect for everyone all of the time. It's not necessarily important that you find the ideal way to use all your strengths but what is important is that you make an effort to become more aware of them and then, that you make an effort to use them (appropriately) as often as you can and in as many situations as you can.

Becoming more aware—or mindfulness—is one of the hottest topics in contemporary psychology, receiving much attention, especially within my specialty area of Positive Psychology. Mindfulness is increasingly being viewed as yet another important coping strategy for living our best lives.

Although defined differently by different people, one of the simplest ways to think about mindfulness is as non-judgemental observation—with curiosity. That is, when we're mindful we observe—with interest but without judgement—our thoughts and feelings, as well as our actions and interactions (with, for example, other people).

Numerous studies over many years now have provided a growing body of evidence supporting the benefits of mindfulness. To cite just one example, researchers from the University of Rochester (in upstate New York) published some impressive results, in 2003, pointing to the relationship between mindfulness and wellbeing and concluding that this relationship came about due to enhanced self-regulation and positive mood states. That is, those who were more mindful were better at managing their own behaviours, acting in ways that were more likely to contribute to wellbeing and, accordingly, they were happier. If that weren't enough a special part of the study that focused on patients with cancer found that increases in mindfulness over time contributed to declines in mood disturbance and stress.

Recent mindfulness research is particularly relevant in the context of this book and should be the cause of great excitement for anyone interested in positive ageing more generally. UK academic psychologist Dr Sophie Sansom led the project investigating whether the well-researched and widely used approach known as Mindfulness Based Stress Reduction (MBSR) could be beneficial for people in the early stages of dementia as a way to offer respite from the difficulties and frustrations experienced with the illness.

In an article published in October 2013 Sansom briefly explained the history of MBSR and then went on to explain that 'for this study we took the [traditional] eight-week programme which has been so successful in other areas and applied it to three groups of people with varying stages of memory problems and dementia in Swindon, Bristol and Exeter . . . we wanted to find out if one; it was possible to teach mindfulness to people with dementia and two; if it improved the quality of life of the sufferer and their primary carer.'

If I were to put on my academic's hat I'd have to say it's too early to confidently state whether or not this intervention has had a significant, positive impact but, as noted earlier, there's enough evidence from other studies with other populations to support the ongoing trialling of mindfulness-based programs with older people. This great quote, from one of the participants in Dr Sansom's research, also provides encouraging support. Mary Corbett, project participant, said:

> We were not worrying about what happened yesterday and what might happen tomorrow but accepting the here and now. We were shown how to let our breathing take over and concentrate on breathing to get the stress away.

And finally, for this chapter anyway, if we recognise and accept that play is helpful and important then how, practicably, can we create more of it in our lives?

To begin with, it might be helpful to define what, exactly, play is! Most experts in this area acknowledge that play is difficult to define because it's an activity—a process—and not a 'thing' or specific outcome. Nevertheless, many have had a go at this challenging task and, according to Stuart Brown, play can be thought of as 'the state of being we experience when we engage in purposeless fun and pleasure.' There's no specific reason for play and there's no specific goal. It is, quite simply, something we should do because it's enjoyable and good for us, in and of itself.

How, then, do we create more of it in our lives? Try some or all of the following and don't forget to have fun with it!

- To begin with, redefine play. If you think it's a waste of time or something that's lacking in utility you're not likely to do it or to keep doing it for very long. Instead, remind yourself of all the benefits that come from having fun and find a way to define play as an essential part of your health and self-care (up there with eating well, getting adequate sleep, and exercising).
- Make it a priority to play every day. It's been said that motivation doesn't last long—but neither does showering, which is why it's recommended we do it regularly! The same could be said for play so find ways to schedule it into your daily routine and reap the rewards of fun and laughter.
- Set aside some time to brainstorm, maybe with your partner, a close friend or relative, and write a list of as many possible ways as you can think of to play.
- Reconnect with play, as recommended by Dr Stuart Brown. Reflect on your past and think of all the times in your life, dating all the way back to childhood, when you enjoyed play, fun and laughter.
- Find other people who are also keen to play. Like many things, play is more fun with others and the good news is there are lots of people out there who enjoy playing. So flick through your address book or contacts list and identify those important people in your life with whom you can enjoy some fun and frivolity.
- Spend time with kids—they're naturally playful and their enthusiasm and energy can rub off on us grown-ups—if we let it!

AND TIME FOR ANOTHER
CONNECTING BIT . . .

Although 'connecting bit' is not necessarily the most beautiful description to use in this context, it consists of two carefully chosen words. Much of what I've written about thus far has been focused on the individual—in most cases, that's 'you', the reader.

And there's good reason for this as you, the reader, are the only one who can take responsibility for and engage in the sorts of healthy and positive behaviours (such as exercise, meditation, optimistic thinking and more) that we know will be helpful. Yet at the same time, it's vitally important to acknowledge that health and happiness and any and all forms of 'success' are not—nor will they ever be—'solo sports'. Rather, happy people have both more and better-quality relationships; healthy people have larger and stronger social support networks that provide them with positive encouragement and buffer them against stress and illness.

With this in mind, in this chapter we look at connections, community, relationships and the importance of all those other people in our lives, as well as us in theirs.

CHAPTER 5

INTERPERSONAL RELATIONSHIPS, CONNECTEDNESS AND BELONGING

'Walking with a friend in the dark is better than walking alone in the light.'

HELEN KELLER

One of the more interesting byways down which I found myself wandering during the course of writing this book, found me chatting away with a sex-worker, on what was for all intents and purposes a normal working day. And this was not just any sex-worker but one who specialised in working with older people (including those with disabilities).

How did this come about? Well, I'm glad you asked because I have a pre-prepared explanation (some might call it an alibi!) that I also shared with my wife at the time.

Around the middle of 2013 I was very flattered to be invited to deliver a keynote presentation at the National Play Up Convention organised by the Arts Health Institute (and my good friend, about whom I've already written, Jean-Paul Bell). At this conference I presented my overarching ideas about positive ageing, which included the topic of this chapter—the importance of relationships and social support. Following my speech I was invited to join a panel where, along with a number of other presenters, we fielded questions from the several hundred-strong audience.

All of the questions were interesting and relevant but one stood out to me and left an indelible mark on my memory because it was both surprising yet obvious. The question was, 'Why, after two days of presentations and workshops within this conference [a conference that focused on the health and wellbeing of older people] has no one mentioned sex?'

We, the 'expert' panel members, looked at each other, smiled (or possibly grimaced) somewhat awkwardly, and then a few of us mumbled some relatively inadequate responses. We then moved on except, in my mind, I didn't move on because I couldn't help but think it was a very important question.

This thought was reinforced just a few weeks later when I stumbled upon an article in my local paper in which an organisation about which I knew nothing was mentioned. The organisation was called 'Touching Base' and in just a few short minutes of reading and researching I discovered who they were and what they did.

Described simply but more than adequately on their website, Touching Base is 'a charitable organisation, based in Sydney Australia, that has been active since October 2000. Touching Base developed out of the need to assist people with disability and sex workers to connect with each other, focusing on access, discrimination, human rights and legal issues and the attitudinal barriers that these two marginalised communities can face.'

In the interests of gaining a better and more complete understanding of the organisation, I scheduled a discussion with Saul Isbister, one of the Founders of Touching Base, which proved both lengthy and fascinating. Among other things, Saul urged me to emphasise two key points. Firstly, Touching Base does not provide the services of sex-workers directly; and secondly, the laws about the provision of sex services vary from state to state and country to country. Here in Australia, however, there are legal ways to access sex-workers in each and every state, and making the public better-informed about such access is one of the primary purposes of Touching Base. In Saul's words, it's about 'equal opportunity' and 'equal access'.

The efforts of Touching Base to assist people with 'disability' have increasingly included the elderly and, following several conversations with Saul, it became obvious to me that it was one of their core beliefs that inspired the organisation's very establish-ment: the belief that just because someone gets old and/or has a form of disability does not, in any way, mean their desires for physical intimacy disappear—nor does it mean they should be denied access to what many would consider a basic human right.

The magazine article to which I referred earlier, and that trig-gered this line of investigation, was entitled 'Senior Moments' and began by asking the intentionally provocative question, 'The elderly don't have sex?'

This question was immediately followed by this answer, 'Carers in nursing homes are seeing otherwise and often butting heads with families and the law over how to deal with it.'

As journalist Peter Munro carefully and thoughtfully pointed out, with an impressive degree of care and compassion and delicacy and balance, 'sex and sexuality do not stop at the front sliding doors, no matter the age of the occupants.' He went on to write about the needs, feelings and desires of older people, as well as the use of inflatable sex dolls, public displays of affection, and simple acts of touch.

Latrobe University sexual health researcher Catherine Barrett is also quoted in the article as saying that 'as a society broadly we don't think of old people as sexual', yet ask anyone working in a nursing home and you'll hear all sorts of stories about residents sneaking into the rooms of other residents; ask many general practitioners who work with this population and you'll also hear concerns about the spread of sexually transmitted illnesses such as Hepatitis C. So, whether we like the idea or not, it's happening!

And why shouldn't it? Of course, by 'it' I don't just mean intercourse. Although for many, intercourse is and will continue to be an important part of life, regardless of age, for others, simply having some form of physical contact is enough. Physical contact is an often-underestimated component of intimacy, and indeed of general health and wellbeing, but there's a considerable body of research that points to the significant benefits of touch.

Believe it or not there's a specialist academic unit, at DePauw University in Indiana, USA, known as the 'Touch and Emotion Lab'. Headed by Dr Matthew Hertenstein, the lab studies physical interactions and displays of emotion. Hertenstein and his team also investigate touch deprivation, which he considers far more common than most people realise.

In a *Huffington Post* article on this topic, written by Diana Spechler, Hertenstein was quoted as saying, 'Most of us, whatever our relationship status, need more human contact than we're getting. Compared with other cultures, we live in a touch-phobic society that's made affection with anyone but loved ones taboo.'

The problem with experiencing touch phobia and contact deprivation is that people are missing out on the measurable health benefits that have been shown to come from physical affection.

The article continues: '"Stimulating touch receptors under the skin can lower blood pressure and cortisol levels, effectively reducing stress," Hertenstein says. One study from the University of North Carolina found that women who hugged their spouse or partner frequently (even for just twenty seconds) had lower blood pressure, possibly because a warm embrace increases oxytocin levels in the brain. Over time, lower blood pressure may decrease a person's risk for heart disease.'

Another researcher in this area, neurologist Shekar Raman, notes that 'a hug, pat on the back, and even a friendly handshake are processed by the reward centre in the central nervous system, which is why they can have a powerful impact on the human psyche, making us feel happiness and joy.'

Older people are still people; and people need other people. The specific needs might change but for many, physical contact is still an important component of a full and flourishing relationship. Which is what this chapter is really all about; the importance of relationships in our lives if we're to enjoy optimum health and wellbeing.

•

In 2009, after more than four decades of research into factors associated with healthy living and longevity, Harvard's George Vaillant was asked in an interview with *The Atlantic* to sum up the most important findings from his 40-plus years of academic work. Without hesitation he responded with, 'The only thing that really matters in life are your relations to other people.'

Although considered rash by some and light and fluffy by others, the basic tenet of Vaillant's summary has been endorsed and supported by many.

Brief mention has already been made of the famous Macarthur Foundation Study of Successful Aging (which ran from 1988 through to 1996), led by John Rowe and involving a team of experts from a range of disciplines. In short, the study identified three components of successful ageing: one, avoiding disease; two, maintaining physical and cognitive activity; and three, engaging fully with life. Notably, this last was then divided into productivity and social support and it's on these aspects that I'd like to focus in this chapter.

In their much-admired text, *Positive Psychology—the Scientific and Practical Explorations of Human Strengths*, co-editors C.R. Snyder and Shane Lopez refer to Rowe's successful ageing research and make the interesting point that social support is most potent when it's mutual; that is, when the support given is balanced by support received.

The editors go on to note that at least two kinds of support are important: one, loving and being loved—socio-emotional support; and two, the provision of assistance to those in need—instrumental support. Close investigation of the Macarthur data reveals that both types of support increased over time and that those people with more positive and supportive relationships experienced markedly less deterioration over that time.

The flip side of this is that a lack of support can result in feelings of loneliness, which can, quite literally, kill! Although (as mentioned earlier) loneliness is almost certainly not as prevalent as many believe, it is still a serious problem and one that's been shown to contribute to markedly poorer health outcomes and quality of life.

In 1970 Lyn Anderson topped the charts with her song, subsequently covered by several famous performers, '(I Never Promised You a) Rose Garden'. Although many have heard this tune and would be familiar with the lyrics, few are aware of the background to this international hit.

Joe South wrote this song in response to Joanne Greenberg's semi-autobiographical novel of the same name (although it was published under the pseudonym Hannah Green), which was also made into a movie. The book was Greenberg's account of her battle with mental illness and her ultimately successful outcome following treatment with a psychoanalyst, Dr Frieda Fromm-Reichmann (immortalised in the film version as Dr Fried). The reason I refer to this here is that Fromm-Reichmann's treatment focused on what she perceived to be Greenberg's loneliness. Mental health, she hypothesised, required social health.

Although psychoanalysis is no longer the dominant approach utilised in psychology and psychiatry (and so Fromm-Reichmann's therapeutic method would not take exactly the same form if it were practised today), the notion that loneliness can have a negative impact on health and wellbeing is still valid and has received more and more support, from many and varied sources, over subsequent decades.

As highlighted by Judith Shulevitz in a fascinating article published in the *New Republic*, 'psychobiologists can now show that loneliness sends misleading hormonal signals, rejiggers the molecules on genes that govern behaviour, and wrenches a slew of other systems out of whack. They have proved that long-lasting loneliness not only makes you sick; it can kill you. Emotional isolation is ranked as [as] high a risk factor for mortality as smoking. A partial list of the physical diseases thought to be caused or exacerbated by loneliness would include Alzheimer's, obesity, diabetes, high blood pressure, heart disease, neurodegenerative diseases, and even cancer—tumours can metastasize faster in lonely people.'

Notably, real loneliness is not synonymous with being alone but more so, should be considered as an internal, subjective experience—an individual can be surrounded by many people but still feel lonely. (If, for example, the individual's perception of these others is that they're not loving or supportive.) Alternatively, an individual can essentially be on his or her own but be perfectly happy. (If the individual believes isolation to be a positive state.)

Although he impressed in many ways, one of the more memorable comments Frank Dearn (the 80-something long-distance runner) made when we talked was that 'fellowship' had always been and continued to be very important in his life. There was absolutely no doubt that although relatively quiet and definitely humble Frank was someone who loved and was loved. His sense of connectedness began with his marriage of more than 45 years, and extended to his church, his activities within Rotary and to his involvement in the Sydney Striders running group, where he was much-liked and revered by all.

Notably, relationships are important in different ways and at different stages of life.

One of the key findings from the Grant Study (or the Harvard Study of Adult Development) was that warm and caring relationships in youth strongly predicted better psychological and physical health later in life. In fact, it's likely that positive relationships are even more important than the many other variables historically considered to be significant.

To make this point more concrete, here's just one specific example from the research findings. Those participants in the study with very high IQs ultimately earned no more income than those with average or slightly above average IQs. Similarly, there were no significant differences in income when those with stronger body types were compared to those with less strong body types and when those with 'working class' fathers were compared to those with 'upper class' fathers.

In contrast, those who were assessed to have a 'warm childhood' with 'good sibling relationships' when young, were found to earn an average of US$51,000 (adjusted to 2009 rates) more a year than those who had poor relationships with their siblings or no siblings at all. The men from 'cohesive' homes made US$66,000 per year more than those from 'unstable' homes. Amazingly, those who described themselves as having warm, caring mothers took home US$87,000 more than those whose mothers were uncaring! And this is when other factors were taken into account.

I should acknowledge that some have criticised the Harvard Grant study for being far from representative (because all the subjects were male and were specifically chosen having been assessed as being healthier and more stable than their peers) so it's questionable whether or not the results can be generalised and applied to other groups of men or the broader population.

However, other studies have been conducted that support these results. To cite one example, the findings of a project in which 'inner-city men' (whose parents were not wealthy) were studied, were very much consistent with those from Harvard. Basically, this study showed that admired fathers, loving mothers and warm friendships were highly predictive of earning a higher income later in life.

And it's not just about predicting income or professional success. Multiple research studies have found that those who grow up in more supportive, loving environments are less likely than those who don't to develop mental health problems or to experience higher levels of depression, anxiety and problems with drugs and alcohol.

In short, there's little doubt that growing up in a loving and caring environment sets one up well for later life. Although we can't go back in time and change the way we were mothered (or raised by our parents), other relationships made throughout our lives are also important and (as has been noted several times so far in this book) it's never too late to work on improving the quality of our relationships and, in doing so, improving the quality of our lives.

Despite the fact that much of the research in this area has been misinterpreted and it's often claimed that those who are married live longer and/or fare better, marriage itself is not necessarily the key. (In many of the relevant studies there are large numbers of people who have been divorced, sometimes multiple times, but who still enjoy the health, wellbeing and longevity benefits that we know are associated with positive relationships.)

Instead, the key to achieving such longevity, it turns out, is not being married per se, but being in loving relationships for long periods of time. To paraphrase one of the key findings from the Harvard Grant study, loving people for a long time is good.

It seems indisputable, then, that having good-quality relationships in your life is healthy and helpful. The next question, however, is why?

Although this is a somewhat more complex question than it might at first appear, there is, at least in the first instance, a relatively simple answer—because it feels good! Most, if not all of us, enjoy loving and being loved and a myriad of studies from a variety of perspectives all support the notion that intimacy is intrinsically linked with positive mental and physical health.

Many years ago, for example, I conducted my doctoral research with patients who were suffering chronic pain; only I wasn't really or directly interested in the chronic pain itself.

What my studies really focused on were the 'dyadic interactions', or the types of responses offered by the 'significant other' (such as a husband, wife, supporter, parent, child) to the person in pain (and, to a lesser extent, the responses offered back to the support person). In short, what we found was that these responses were significant determinants of pain, levels of distress experienced and levels of functioning.

More specifically, the patients whose significant others were deemed to respond to their displays of pain with 'punishing responses' (getting angry and abusive or criticising the person for not doing more, for example) tended to report higher levels of pain intensity and markedly more distress. Conversely, those patients whose partners responded with 'overly solicitous responses' (such as taking over chores, encouraging them to rest or doing everything for them) reported less distress but far more dysfunction. Finally, significant others who responded with 'supportive responses' (empathy combined with encouragement) were far more likely to function well and with less distress, despite ongoing pain.

In summary then, the nature and quality of a relationship and the responses that occur within that relationship are very important as they can ultimately contribute to higher or lower levels of mental and physical health and functioning.

Interestingly, much of the marital therapy or couples research has (until relatively recently) focused almost exclusively on the 'unhelpful' or negative behaviours or interactions, believing that if we can just understand these destructive interpersonal behaviours, we can then try to remedy them. While this is not a completely irrational approach, there's another—very different—one, which has been advocated for quite a few decades now and which has seen increasing scientific support. This approach proffers the idea that focusing on what goes right is almost certainly more useful than focusing on what goes wrong.

Several decades ago, for example, Dr John Gottman began his research into couples, bucking what at the time was the most dominant trend of studying only those couples who were low on satisfaction or reported high distress within their marriages and trying to understand what was going wrong. As just noted, the popular assumption at the time was that if we could better understand what was going wrong, we'd be able to fix the problem and so improve these relationships.

However, as we now know from the last few decades of research into Positive Psychology, if you take something that's bad and fix it, you don't necessarily get good! An absence of depression, for example, does not necessarily equate to the presence of happiness.

Gottman preceded the Positive Psychology movement by quite a few years and, in what now seems a prescient and brilliant move, he thought to ask not what was going wrong with distressed couples but what was going right with happy and satisfied couples.

This is important because, as noted above, the lack of a healthy and satisfying relationship need not bring about an early death; one can continue to work on improving one's relationship and/ or search for new and more satisfying relationships to gain the benefits of loving and being loved over a long period of time.

So what can we learn from Gottman's 40-plus years of research? In short, his findings showed that those couples reporting higher levels of health and wellbeing (and especially marital satisfaction) experienced significantly more positive than negative interactions within their relationships, which is in keeping with my overarching belief in this chapter.

Earlier in this book I referred to Barbara Fredrickson's research and, notably, to her famous 'positivity ratio' (the critical range for a person's positive to negative emotions) in which those people who reported and who were assessed to be thriving had a higher proportion of positive to negative emotions in their lives. The positivity ratio that resulted from Fredrickson's research was three to one. Amazingly, the ratio discovered from Gottman's completely unrelated research was very similar, at about five to one. What this means is that for every negative interaction these satisfied couples had (and they did have some negative experiences), they created at least five positive interactions. In fact, some research suggests happy couples argue and disagree just as much as unhappy couples but they make up much better and more quickly, and fill the time in between with significantly more positive experiences.

John Gottman has, over the years, written (or co-written) more than 40 books and published almost 200 papers and almost all of these works have avoided the emphasis common to most other marital or couples experts, which was to focus on what's wrong with relationships and then try to fix them. Instead, Gottman and his team of researchers have shown that it's not just how couples fight that matters but more importantly, how they make up!

This theme of looking at the things that go right within relationships is something that interests me and that I've seen time and time again in my clinical psychology—and more recently executive coaching—practice. In all areas where relationships matter—and let's face it, relationships matter in all areas—disagreements occur, but the most loving and happy partners and the most successful leaders and managers (when we look at this within an organisational or occupational domain) are far better at and devote much more time to reconciling after a fight or some sort of negative experience.

This was especially evident in Simon, a client of mine who came to see me due to concerns about his relationship with his teenage daughter. Simon dearly loved each of his three children, including his adolescent daughter, but was struggling to cope with the changes she was going through and the way they were being expressed in certain behaviours and mood swings.

Now any parent of a teenager will probably relate to this—and especially the parent of a teenage girl—but the fact it's common and arguably even 'normal' doesn't necessarily make it any easier to cope with and Simon was worried that his and his daughter's relationship was suffering irreparable damage (not to mention the effect and strain it was having on his wife and two other children).

Eventually, though, it turned out that one relatively simple strategy managed to radically change the nature and quality of their interactions and, accordingly, their relationship. Following some collaborative research, Simon and I both came to the conclusion that parenting teenagers generally, and fathering a teenage girl specifically, would inevitably have its challenges and include at least some disagreements and arguments. Trying to eliminate these completely or expecting not to have any disagreements would lead to frustration and disappointment and almost certainly end in failure.

At the same time, however, we agreed there had to be a better way. As is my wont (as a coach, therapist and everyday person) my starting point for finding a solution to this problem was the reality of the situation, which meant accepting at least some friction in the parent-teenager relationship. From this point Simon and I discussed how best to manage such friction and importantly, having discussed some of Gottman's research together, how to make up as quickly as possible in between disagreements and how to fill the gaps between disagreements with as much positivity as possible.

As a result of several discussions and some thinking time, Simon came back to me with the following great ideas:

- He would make an effort to apologise as quickly as possible whenever and wherever relevant.
- Each episode of disagreement would be contained and both would agree (as best they could) not to hold grudges or to

extend the length of time either person was upset beyond the reasonable.

- Both Simon and his daughter drew up lists of three to five things they'd like the other person to do during disagreements and they would each try their best to adhere to these requests (e.g. to listen to the other person before making decisions, to try to empathise).

- At least once each week they'd have 'special time' together, with no gadgets or devices, when they would be totally present and available to listen to the other person.

- Simon would also make a concerted effort to show interest in the things his daughter was increasingly becoming interested in so they'd have more in common about which they could talk and connect.

- And probably most importantly, Simon made a mental note to more consciously be on the lookout for times when his daughter was doing things right, when she was engaging in positive and desirable behaviours; he was going to make sure he caught her when she was doing things right not just when she was doing things wrong!

All of this achieved two positive outcomes: the extent to which both parties became upset during and immediately after disagreements was significantly reduced and the extent to which they enjoyed each other's company was significantly increased. Simon and his daughter still, notably, argued and had some unpleasant times together but such instances were far less frequent and seemed far less significant within the context of greater positivity.

This theory isn't just about parenting teenage girls, though. The same basic principle applies to anyone in any relationship, whether with a child, a partner, a friend or a colleague.

When I happened to mention this research, and the outcome of my sessions with Simon, to a friend who was struggling with her own stressful relationship she reacted with amazement and reported experiencing something of an epiphany. It turns out her mother was ageing and going through a very difficult period of adjustment. Her health and level of functioning were deteriorating and, secondary to this, her mood was suffering. My friend Jane expressed her distress associated with having fewer and fewer positive experiences with her mother.

But in the light of the aforementioned research and case study, Jane smiled and noted she could now see a better way. Very much like Simon, Jane realised she had to accept that her mother was changing and that accordingly their relationship would change. She probably had to accept that her mother would increasingly face both physical and cognitive difficulties and challenges bringing along a number of negatives and a certain degree of distress. But, and here's where the similarities with Simon come in, Jane also realised there would be a plentiful supply of opportunities in between these negative situations and problems in which to laugh and smile, to enjoy each other and to appreciate life. Jane was determined to highlight and celebrate these positive moments and to contain and minimise the negative ones as best she could.

And this is all entirely consistent with the work of another pioneering researcher, Shelly Gable. In 2004, Gable and her colleagues at the University of California and the University of Rochester completed a series of four studies focusing on the consequences of different types of interpersonal reactions when good things happen. Just over 150 men and women were recruited into the study and they were given a number of booklets within which they were asked to record a number of things each and every night.

One of the key variables they were asked to record was 'the most important positive event or issue of the day'. In addition, participants were also asked to note how much they let others know about the event or issue and, notably, a new scale was developed specifically for the study to determine each person's perception of their partners' responses to the sharing of positive events.

In short, the first two studies effectively showed that talking about positive experiences with others is associated with increases in daily positive feelings as well as general happiness and wellbeing.

Although both are important findings, the second is much more interesting in the context of this book and vastly more significant in terms of the implications it has for positive relationships. The benefits of talking about positive experiences, as seen in the study, were significantly enhanced when the person hearing about those experiences responded in a way that was described as 'active and constructive' (as opposed to 'passive and destructive'). Further, the participants in close relationships (that were more prevalent amongst the active and constructive responses) reported much higher levels of relationship wellbeing (including intimacy and marital satisfaction).

Let me give you a concrete example. When I received notification that the publishers wanted to proceed with this book I immediately told the most important person in my life—my wife. Now thankfully I can say I have a fantastic marital relationship and a wife who naturally responds in the ideal way identified in Gable's research. So when I told her my good news she actively responded with enthusiasm, joy, pride and excitement. She asked me what the book was about, when the manuscript was due and many other questions, all of which showed me she was pleased for me and genuinely interested in my new project. This active and constructive response was close to perfect but unfortunately such a response to good news is not as common as we might like to think.

Imagine for a minute that my relationship was not as strong and that a different, hypothetical wife was more prone to passive, destructive responses. If this were the case her response to such news might have been something more like: 'Oh, that's interesting, dear; can you take the rubbish out and then help clean up the kitchen so we can start to get dinner ready?' (Passive.)

Or even, 'Great. [Said with a sarcastic tone.] You're already so busy we hardly ever see you and now you'll just be working longer hours, on something that won't make us any money, and I'll have to do even more work around the house and with the kids!' (Active and destructive.)

Not surprisingly, these types of responses do not lead to good-quality relationships, but the good news is we can all learn—or we can all get help to learn—from Gottman, Gable and others, applying the findings of their many wonderful studies to our real-world relationships. Before looking at some practical strategies, however, let me just refer to one other fascinating stream of research.

Just a few years ago, in 2009, a group of researchers from the University of Arizona and the Washington University in St Louis conducted a study together to which they gave the fascinating title 'Eavesdropping on happiness: well-being is related to having less small talk and more substantive conversations.' And they did, quite literally, eavesdrop on interpersonal interactions by using a wonderful piece of gadgetry—a digital audio recorder that 'unobtrusively tracks real-world behaviour by periodically recording snippets of ambient sounds while participants go about their daily lives.' In other words, they overcame one of the greatest obstacles faced by much social science research and actually listened to people and their conversations in the real world, rather to than those people's recollections of their conversations or to conversations in an artificial setting like a laboratory.

Amazingly, the researchers gathered more than 23,000 waking recordings, which equated to approximately 300 per participant. Several of the researchers then had the unenviable job of listening to each and every recording and coding the conversations based on whether the person was alone or not, and whether the conversation consisted of 'small talk' or 'substantive conversation'. (I should explain that small talk was defined by the researchers as 'uninvolved or banal interaction in which only trivial information was exchanged', whereas substantive conversation was defined as being more involved and meaningful.)

As is almost always the case, it's the data or results section of the paper where things get interesting. Consistent with a number of other studies the research confirmed that greater wellbeing was positively associated with spending less time alone and more time talking to others. But not all examples of 'talking to others' were equally beneficial; better wellbeing was much more likely to be associated with having less small talk and more meaningful conversations. Specifically, the happiest participants spent 25 per cent less time alone and 70 per cent more time talking! They also had approximately one third as much small talk and twice as many substantive conversations. These are big differences that lead to important health and wellbeing benefits.

To sum up, then, we know that loneliness is far from ideal if one wants to live a long and healthy life. In contrast, those who have more and better quality relationships live longer, healthier and happier lives; they're more connected and have a greater sense of belonging; they have more positive and meaningful interactions with more people and although they still argue and disagree with family and friends (like all of us), they remedy the situation by making up much better and faster.

Of course, any of us can do these things—or learn to do them. I'd strongly suggest we all work hard to do so, because (as I hope I've made clear over the last few thousand words) mastering these skills will contribute significantly to improving health, happiness and life.

So here are a few practical tips to boost the quality of your interactions with others:

- Keep a diary or journal of the positive experiences you enjoy every day and week and then, when appropriate (preferably at least once each week, although the more often the better), share these positive experiences with a loved one, family member or friend.
- Although quality is obviously important, so too is quantity, so make an effort to have more interactions with more people more often.

- Ensure, whenever possible, that the bulk of your interactions are positive and meaningful.
- Catch people when they do things right—that is, look for opportunities to reinforce and reward others for their good actions and deeds.
- See the best in others—that is, make a concerted effort to focus on other people's strengths, positive attributes and qualities rather than on their faults and weaknesses.
- Until proved otherwise, assume the best about and believe the best in others—withhold judgement as much as possible. (Unless, obviously, you have good evidence and/or reason to form a negative opinion.)
- Be the person that brings positivity and enthusiasm, love and compassion to each and every interaction.
- Respect and accept others for who and what they are, rather than seeing them for who they're not or what you think they 'should' be.
- Acknowledge and talk about disagreements, accept that arguments will occur, but take steps quickly to forgive and make up, resolving any conflicts as soon as is reasonably possible.
- Look for opportunities to laugh and have fun, to joke and to enjoy life with others!

Finally, it's worth emphasising (in case I've not made it clear already) that the benefits of relationships don't just come from engaging positively with those closest to us (such as husbands and wives, boyfriends and girlfriends, children, parents or other relatives) but also from those in the broader context of our lives.

Feeling as though one belongs to a community has also been found to promote health and wellbeing in numerous ways.

Socialising with friends, for example, significantly increases our chances of maintaining brain- and memory function as we age. Harvard University's School of Public Health found this after surveying more than 16,000 people over a six-year period (1998 through to 2004). And the results were pretty amazing.

People with the highest levels of social interaction were far more likely to retain higher levels of cognitive function—that is, their brains continued to work better for longer. And what was especially impressive is that the findings were just as strong for those considered to be at high risk of dementia (such as those with lower levels of education and more vascular conditions like high blood pressure, diabetes or a history of stroke).

Importantly, these findings have been supported by other sizeable studies, including one that covered more than 2000 women aged over 78 and assessed, several times, over a four-year period. Again, the researchers found that women with large social networks were less likely to develop dementia than those who were more isolated.

Although from the evidence seen so far we can quite confidently assert that social contact provides important mental and physical health benefits it's important to note that explanations as to how this works are more hypothetical. That is, we know that social interaction helps but we're a little less sure about *how* it helps.

Nevertheless, most experts in this area agree that the benefits are most likely to come about as a result of one or more of the following:

- Regular social contact—this is likely to promote and to be associated with more healthy behaviours (such as walking and generally keeping active). In addition, regular social contact is more likely to make it easier to access medical help if and when necessary (this could occur due to friends encouraging others to see a doctor if they notice concerning signs or symptoms and/or due to offers and provision of transport to actually get to a medical surgery or hospital).
- Interpersonal and group interactions—these have been shown to reduce stress (those with higher levels of socialising are less likely to experience the range of stress-related illnesses).
- Social activities—these are, more often than not, emotionally and intellectually stimulating, which we know contributes to the fostering of better neuronal connections and even nerve growth in the brain.

So the question now becomes not, should I connect more with others and find ways to interact? but instead, how can I become more socially active, because it's vitally important for my health and wellbeing?

And I'm glad you asked that question because following on from suggestions made in other parts of this book and in response to those of AMAC (The Voice of Americans 50+), I have a few answers:

- If you normally wait for others to reach out, pick up the phone first and propose a date to meet.
- Make a difference in someone's life. Explore some of the many volunteer opportunities available, from wielding tools

to sprucing up affordable housing to mentoring a child or businessperson.

- Consider re-joining the workforce. Besides bolstering your finances, a job can offer opportunities to connect with others.
- Harness the warmer side of technology. E-mail and telephones extend our reach around the world. Libraries and senior centres may offer free online time and may even help you set up a free e-mail account.
- Find like-minded individuals through organisations or hobbies that interest you. Local newspapers are a good source of information.
- Return to the classroom. Learn a new skill, brush up on an old one or pursue a passion. Local colleges and adult education centres offer up a variety of new experiences, from learning to sail to studying art history to finding out how to make the perfect crème brûlée.

Connecting with others and finding or creating a sense of community is such an important issue that we'll return to it, in a slightly different way, in the final chapter of the book. But for now, and as we bring this chapter to an end, remember Marcel Proust's words: '. . . let us be grateful to the people who make us happy, they are the charming gardeners who make our souls blossom.'

SOMETIMES THINGS GO BAD . . .

As just noted in Chapter Five, the people in our lives can be loving, caring, supportive and encouraging and, when this happens, good-quality relationships result that can have incredibly positive effects on our health, happiness and success in life generally. We all need, and benefit from, help at times.

However as most of us are well aware, not all relationships are nourishing or healing—or at least not all will end well. Most of us have had some experience of being harmed, wronged, cheated or even physically hurt—and some of us have done the harming, hurting or cheating.

Accordingly, we all have people in our lives that contribute to negative (and sometimes extremely damaging) feelings, such as hate, anger and regret. As with all other areas of life, we have choices in how we deal with such emotions: we can deny and ignore the issues, hoping they just go away or somehow magically disappear; or we can face up to them, deal with them constructively and, ideally, do what we can to turn pain into something from which we can learn, to change distress into growth.

Not surprisingly, it's the latter approach that I advocate and I'll be explaining more in the next chapter.

CHAPTER 6
DEALING WITH REGRETS AND RESOLVING OLD HURTS

'Do not regret growing older,
it's a privilege denied to many.'
(UNKNOWN)

If I were going to write a list of the top few 'killers' it would be hard to go past alcohol and cigarettes. If I then extended this list to include psychological and social variables I'd probably then go to loneliness (as already referred to quite a few times); after that, one particularly destructive emotion comes to mind: anger!

In 1996 Todd Miller and colleagues published a meta-analytical review of research linking hostility and physical health in the highly regarded *Psychological Bulletin*. Meta-analysis is a much-valued approach as it brings together a variety of data, combining and contrasting results from different studies. Compared to individual studies that are of course important in other ways, these meta-analyses allow investigators to look for and potentially identify patterns among and across different studies. Ultimately, this allows academics to more powerfully estimate the real effects and power of interventions or relationships.

Miller's analysis included 45 different studies and the results clearly showed that even when other factors were taken into account, hostility was an independent risk factor for coronary heart disease. In short, holding on to past hurts and allowing anger to fester and grow will, ultimately, kill.

During one of my reconnaissance visits to a local lifestyle village, I spent a wonderful half hour or so chatting to a woman named Nancy. Nancy was born in London, came to Australia as a toddler, is currently 85 years old and smiled throughout each and every minute of our informal interview. The details of Nancy's past are not relevant here, but suffice to say she'd had her fair share of tough times and challenges and had faced more than enough adversity.

The reason I'm relating a story about Nancy here is not because of her past, though—it's because of her present. When I asked her to describe a typical day she noted, with a lovely, genuine smile, that she couldn't really take part in many of the activities the village organised and in which her friends participated, but she loved to watch and to share their stories and, most of all, to hear their laughter as they engaged in the scheduled leisure activities of the day.

In the back of my mind I was curious to ask how she felt about 'missing out' but before I could do so she beat me to the punch, saying, 'You know, I used to be one of the most active residents here; involved in anything and everything I could get involved in. But over the last few years I've found I just can't do what I used to do so now I'm just happy to watch.'

Nancy's story is a great example of what's been discovered in a series of fascinating research studies; that the ability to accept what cannot be changed is key to happiness in old age, after declines in functioning or loss of independence. Although ageing need not necessarily equate to the physical and mental deterioration and decline too often portrayed by the media (as previously noted), it is important to be realistic and the reality for all of us is that at some point we will experience at least some loss of functioning and/or mental acuity.

Believing this 'won't' or 'shouldn't' happen will only lead to frustration and disappointment; believing that all areas of performance and living will be maintained at or near to the highest level will only lead to feelings of being let down and depression.

In June 2013, when I was in the very early stages of writing this book, I was very pleased to discover an article by a group of Australian psychologists based at Deakin University in Victoria. In their study, Jaclyn Broadbent and her colleagues looked at the relationship between perceived control and eight areas of life satisfaction in just over 100 older adults (defined as 65 years and above) living in the community as well as another 100 living in residential aged-care facilities.

Not surprisingly, higher levels of perceived control were correlated with higher levels of life satisfaction and happiness; but what was also discovered was the mediating role played by acceptance. That is, as actual control declined the role of acceptance increased and buffered or protected individuals against a decline in satisfaction and wellbeing. So, in short, it's important to believe you're in control of yourself and of your life, but it's also important to accept that some things, ultimately, are beyond our control.

This finding, I strongly suspect, applies not just to loss of or changes in functioning, but also to aspects of our past over which, obviously, we have no control.

What we can learn from all of this is that acceptance and forgiveness are crucial to living a long, healthy and happy life. We've all been wronged—or at least we all believe we've been wronged—but it's in no one's interest to allow this to ruin years and years of what could be filled with good relationships.

I'll never forget my father talking about how his father and uncle didn't speak for the last few decades (yes, decades!) of their lives because of a disagreement, the topic of which neither of them could even remember. And along similar lines is this great quote, attributed to the Buddha, which I stumbled upon many years ago now: 'Holding on to anger is like grasping a hot coal with the intent of throwing it at someone else; you are the one getting burned.'

Further to this, one of the most interesting books I've ever read was called *Beyond Revenge: The Evolution of the Forgiveness Instinct*, written by a Professor of Psychology based in Miami. In it, Michael McCullough reviews large amounts of research from social and evolutionary psychology and essentially concludes that anger and revenge are normal (and at times appropriate) human responses, but that so too is forgiveness. In fact according to McCullough forgiveness of others allows us to then get on with each other and to live long and healthy lives despite having previously been wronged or harmed.

In the introductory chapter, McCullough sets the scene by explicitly stating that he wrote his book for two groups of people: those who want to see human nature for what it really is, and those who want to make the world a better place. He goes on to argue that the goals of these two groups are intimately connected and that to achieve them one must learn what he believes to be three simple truths about revenge and forgiveness:

1. The desire for revenge is a built-in feature of human nature.
2. The capacity for forgiveness is a built-in feature of human nature.
3. To make the world a more forgiving, less vengeful, place we need to stop trying to change human nature and focus, instead, on changing the world.

As with all good scientists, McCullough makes an effort to explain the logic behind his book's theory and, in so doing, provides the following definition of revenge:

> Revenge . . . is any attempt to harm someone or some group of people in response to feeling that oneself has been harmed by that other person or group, whereby the act of harming that person or group is *not* designed to repair the harm, to stop it from occurring or continuing in the immediate confrontation, or to produce material gain.

Again, unsurprisingly, he proffers that revenge is a problem, but he also points out, 'the desire for revenge is one thing; acting on it is another.' This is very important to note as it highlights that when we think of revenge as being a problem (as most of us do), what we're really thinking about are the problematic acts of aggression and violence (such as, in the worst-case situations, murder and war) that often stem from a desire for revenge.

I think we'd all agree that we should be doing whatever we

can to curb violence and aggression. Taking 'an eye for an eye', as the old saying goes, just leaves everybody blind and achieves little or nothing of value in the process.

Yet if McCullough is right, and there's no doubt he's done his research on this topic, then we might be fighting a losing battle (if you'll excuse the possibly inappropriate metaphor) trying to change human nature. Because it can be argued that the feelings associated with a desire for revenge are 'natural' and even, in some contexts, appropriate.

Anthropology, the comparative study of human societies and cultures and their development, provides numerous examples of how people have been killing other people for as long as we can determine. Most anthropologists also agree that the avenging of killings with murder is a universal phenomenon and some argue that it is even associated with a form of social organisation. Specifically, it's hypothesised that a wrong can be righted by a sanctioned wrong ending and consequently the prospect of ongoing and escalating violence or aggressive action.

Over time, however, as societies advanced, many introduced sanctions and controls to ensure revenge-motivated homicides or acts of aggression are managed in some way. But many societies also recognise that revenge might, in some way, be part of a solution.

McCullough cites a plethora of fascinating research studies (that are valid and well-supported with evidence) putting forward an entirely plausible notion that might be called 'controlled revenge as adaptive'. Revenge, for example, could be considered adaptive if it deters aggressors from repeating their acts of aggression. Just as importantly, if not more so, revenge could serve an adaptive function by warning off potential wrongdoers before they actually commit an act of violence or harm, acting, therefore, as a preventative.

Putting all of this together, McCullough's key message is that we should be trying to learn from and take 'the best bits' of revenge while ensuring, at the same time, we protect against the worst. To do this, he argues that we not only try to understand what circumstances and conditions increase the likelihood of revenge serving a useful role in our lives but, more importantly, we learn the practical steps necessary to enhance forgiveness.

•

One of the wonderful aspects of the longitudinal studies to which I've already referred within this book (such as the Harvard Grant Study) is that their findings have provided us with a perspective on life over many, many decades (rather than just a cross-sectional view at one fixed point in time). This is important because the meaning and value of certain situations and experiences can change.

Although hard to fathom now, there was a time when people such as Hitler and Stalin were considered by some to be 'great leaders'. Clearly, with hindsight, that judgement has changed. In the same way, what might have been considered unpleasant for some individuals can, over time, be viewed as useful. In his book about the Harvard Grant Study, *Triumphs of Experiences*, George Vaillant writes, 'as in the inflammations and fevers of physical illness, what looks like trouble may be the very process by which healing takes place. As we become better able to endure life's slings and arrows, our coping mechanisms mature.'

More and more research is pointing to the same conclusion – that what goes right is more important than what goes wrong; and even what goes wrong can be important in a positive way if it's 'used' constructively.

This leads into some related and relatively recent research, from which it's been found that although undoubtedly unpleasant at the time negative life events can, in many instances, come to be viewed as helpful or useful if they lead in some way towards learning, maturation or the gaining of strength and/or wisdom.

Although one can conclude from many of the scientific findings that early-life successes, rather than failures, are predictive of later-life mental and physical health it can also be asserted that what people do with troubled childhoods or negative early-life events—that is, how they respond to, interpret and ultimately make meaning of them—is equally important in predicting long-term quality of life.

The basic idea that positive changes can eventuate from suffering and distress is not new; there are references to a range of similar concepts dating back thousands of years. Ancient Buddhist, Hebrew and other texts have, in a variety of ways, suggested that pain and negative life events can be positively transforming ultimately. In fact it could be argued that attempts to understand and make sense of human suffering and its relationship to living have formed the heart and soul of many of the theories of some of our greatest writers, poets and philosophers.

In the last twenty or so years, however, there's been a much greater and more formal academic focus on what's come to be called 'post-traumatic growth', as the interests of many researchers have shifted from the negative to the positive; as opposed to just investigating where and what goes wrong and what leads to distress and dysfunction, researchers have moved towards trying to understand how and why people survive and thrive, who does well and what it is that helps them to do well.

What I'm referring to, then, is the relatively recent acknowledgement of a positive psychological change that can come about as a direct or indirect result of negative and often challenging life circumstances. Earlier this year (in 2013) Dalnim Cho and a colleague from the University of Connecticut published a comprehensive review of 'growth following trauma'. They studied almost 70 publications and considered several models of growth as well as the factors that contribute to growth.

Now before continuing it's important to state, as Cho and Park did in their paper, 'the aftermath of highly stressful events differs from person to person.' Having noted this, however, they then went on to conclude that whether the negative event was a cancer diagnosis, sexual assault or the death of a loved one; whether it was exposure to an incident of terror or something entirely different, 'many people report positive growth following adversity.'

An important question, then, is why does this growth occur? Understanding the underlying processes would almost certainly help us to help others to maximise growth following trauma.

Cho and Park examined several theories, including the following:

- Traumatic events affect people's assumptive worlds: following significant negative life events people change the way they think about themselves and the world around them.
- We gain strength through suffering: along the lines of the 'no pain no gain' motto.

- Survivors become resistant to subsequent trauma in a similar way to those who've been vaccinated in medicine becoming resistant to certain illnesses.
- Existential re-evaluation occurs following trauma via a process of 'meaning making'.
- Bonds with significant others are strengthened by traumatic events: in sharing problems we can actually build more positive relationships with others.

These various theories are almost certainly not mutually exclusive and the presence or utilisation of specific coping strategies within each one is also very important. Although many of these coping strategies have been referred to in a number of the studies conducted in this area, the most commonly cited ones, considered to be the most important, include:

- cognitive reappraisal—thinking about events in more helpful ways
- developing an openness to new experiences—seeing new events as interesting as opposed to entirely negative
- striving for a higher level of self-control
- developing a belief that other people and the world generally are benevolent
- having a greater willingness to engage in emotional expression (talking to others about how one's feeling, for example)
- spirituality or the belief that there's some greater purpose or meaning
- play.

The good news is that all of these strategies can be taught and, as a result, we can all learn to think back to past life events—even negative and painful ones—and feel less pain and even gain a sense that we have, as a result of such events, become wiser or stronger, better or even happier.

How?

I invite you to begin by giving some serious consideration to the following:

- Reflect on the situation or event and ask yourself:
  o Did I survive?
  o Was it really that bad?
  o Was there any real, permanent damage?

The goal of this first step is to ensure you have the events on which you're focusing in perspective. Even if the situation was 'very bad' there are still some important questions you can ask yourself, such as: What did it mean to me? What, if anything, did I learn? Did I gain anything from this situation? Were any of my relationships strengthened? Am I thinking about myself as a victim in this situation or as a survivor or maybe even a thriver?

Now you've taken the first step, here are some more tips and strategies:

- What did you actually do to cope in the situation or with the stressor? Have you fully acknowledged these efforts? Have you given yourself a literal or metaphorical pat on the back for doing what you did?

- As a result of this event and/or any subsequent associated changes is it possible your life is in some way better? Is it possible in any way that your future is better or brighter? Could you look at yourself as now being wiser, more mature, stronger or in any way improved?
- Has the pain and suffering you experienced given you knowledge or the ability to cope more effectively with future events and challenges? If so, do you properly acknowledge and see the utility in this?
- Often, trauma and stress challenge us to make moral or ethical decisions; was this the case for you and, if so, have you subsequently become clearer about your values or your priorities?

Please note that this section is not intended to imply, in any way, that trauma or stress are good things or that we should only look 'positively' on such life events. To do so would be not only absurd but almost certainly unhelpful. Rather, by raising the idea of post-traumatic growth my hope is that you'll give at least some thought to what can potentially be gained from negative situations, and how difficult events can be used and built upon to limit future adversity or manage it more effectively when it is unavoidable.

In her wonderfully written and fantastically practical book, *The How of Happiness*, Sonja Lyubomirsky acknowledges that forgiveness is an important part of happiness because, in short, we've all been wronged and if we don't forgive we'll all go on experiencing grief and anger (which achieves little, if anything, of value). In doing so she offers the following simple but effective strategies for practising forgiveness:

- Recall a time when you were forgiven; when somebody else paid you the courtesy of forgiving a wrong you'd committed (whether intentionally or unintentionally). Bring to mind what it felt like and imagine extending or sharing that gift with someone else.

- Seek and/or ask forgiveness of others. Apologise to someone you've wronged, either in person or, if more appropriate, via a letter or phone call or some other means. By seeking forgiveness you can (as with the previous point) benefit and gain a greater understanding of how the process works and of how beneficial it can be. The idea is that this will increase your ability to forgive others.

- If you're really struggling to forgive someone else then just begin by imagining what it might be like if you were able to forgive them; you're not actually forgiving yet, but just taking a first, small step by using your imagination. Having suggested this strategy to a number of clients I've found that it makes it much easier, then, to take the next step towards real forgiveness.

- Try to feel even the smallest sliver of empathy for the other person; the person who you believe has wronged you. Without necessarily condoning or agreeing with their behaviour, or excusing or even forgetting what they've done, try to find a perspective from which you can understand why they might have done what they did. Once you've found this, imagine it expanding, growing and becoming more significant.

- Learn about, practise and utilise other strategies that will minimise worry and rumination. Thinking over and over again about something (and it can be anything) that's having a negative impact is rarely helpful and especially in this context (where there may be little you can do to change the situation or force the other person to take remedial action), it may be best to focus on other, more constructive and positive endeavours and topics.

• Finally, one of the best cures for unhappiness is happiness and, similarly, one of the best cures for bitterness and acrimony is kindness, generosity and good will. So do good for others, because ultimately forgiveness is something that will benefit you!

If you're reading this then I'm pretty confident in assuming that . . . you're alive! And if you're alive then there's still time to avoid regrets. Many of us arrive at our later years upset that we've not accomplished something, completed something or in some way or other lived the life we would have liked to have lived. But as just noted it's not too late and it's especially not too late to avoid or resolve some of the more common regrets.

A few years ago an Australian nurse published a book based on her years of experience working in palliative care. In *The Top Five Regrets of the Dying*, Bronnie Ware recorded the thoughts and comments of those in their final days. No one mentioned wishing that they'd worked harder or longer—and I don't believe anyone mentioned wishing they'd gone bungee jumping! What many of the patients did mention, however, were the following regrets:

1. I wish I'd had the courage to live a life true to myself, not the life others expected of me. (This was the most common regret of all.)
2. I wish I hadn't worked so hard.

3. I wish I'd had the courage to express my feelings.
4. I wish I'd stayed in touch with my friends.
5. I wish that I had let myself be happier.

And the great thing about this list is that all of it, or almost all of it, can be reversed or undone—no matter how old you are right now!

Admittedly, we can't go back in time and change each and every aspect of the past. But we can start today to live differently and create new and better futures because each and every one of these points can be used to motivate us to live better lives.

We can, for example, start living a life that's true to ourselves any day and any time. We can start working less (if this is relevant) and playing more. We can express ourselves and our feelings more and we can get in touch or reconnect with old friends and family. Finally, we can (and indeed should) allow ourselves to be happier—because if not now then when?

In fact, that's what this book is essentially about. It's about making the most of our lives from here on in. No one, no matter what age we are, can change the past; but we can learn from the past and use those lessons to enjoy a better future. Whether that future will be one day, one week, one month, one year or (hopefully) longer, none of us know. But it doesn't really matter. As much as we want to plan for the future (and we do) it's vitally important to enjoy this very moment—starting now—and continue to do so for each and every moment that follows!

EVERY CLOUD HAS A SILVER LINING . . .

There's not one of us who can completely avoid pain and suffering, but all of us can learn from experiences of distress and difficulty and, ideally, find ways to grow and improve ourselves from the lessons we learn in or after these situations. The reality is, however, that although we all develop as we age, some do so far more effectively than others.

Interestingly, and not all that surprisingly, those who develop and mature in more healthy ways tend to live longer and better. The good news is that plenty of research has led to a strong understanding of what this process of maturation is, how it works, and what approaches towards it work best.

So read the next chapter to learn more about how growth and development are part of positive ageing and, notably, what each and every one of you can do to maximise your chances of achieving the most desirable stages of maturity.

CHAPTER 7

MATURATION, WISDOM, PERSONAL IDENTITY AND REDEFINING WHO I AM

'For the unlearned, old age is winter; for the learned, it is the season of the harvest.'
HASIDIC SAYING

I'm not exaggerating when I write that I have, literally, seen more than a thousand clients during my years as a clinical psychologist (therapist) and more recently, as an executive coach. If you include all the people I've spoken to before, during and after conferences and events at which I've presented (or even just attended) then the number would most likely be in the tens of thousands.

Many of these people have shared with me some interesting and memorable stories. A few in particular really stand out and I'd like to share with you one I heard a few years ago, involving a client I'll call Peter.

Peter was in his early fifties and was, for all intents and purposes, relatively healthy and happy. He was 'successful' in most meanings of the word, in that he had achieved much professionally (becoming a partner in a highly regarded and internationally renowned professional services firm) and financially (he owned a very nice house in a very nice suburb of one of the best and most liveable cities in the world, Sydney). He was also happily married (with two healthy children, both of whom were faring well socially and academically). On the surface, there was little to indicate anything except that Peter had a great life. But under the surface, as I discovered relatively quickly once he commenced a course of coaching, this was not the case—Peter was terrified!

It turned out that although he was very good at what he did professionally and was highly respected by both his peers and clients, Peter had grown tired of his career. He didn't 'hate' it per se but he'd become pretty bored of it in recent years and found it increasingly less satisfying, pleasurable, meaningful and challenging. He told me, without any hint of arrogance or boastfulness, that he'd achieved pretty much everything he wanted to achieve and had begun to consider the next stage of his life—but he had absolutely no idea what this would be!

Like many successful professionals, Peter had worked hard at high school to secure the necessary (high) leaving certificate mark, and then he'd worked even harder at university to ensure he achieved the best grades so he'd be offered not just any job, but a job in one of the 'Big Four' (the largest and most respected firms in the country). Peter succeeded in doing so, but he didn't stop there; he then had to keep working just as hard as he had through high school and university (if not harder), to prove himself among all the other high achievers so that he could then progress to the 'partner track'. This he did and then—well, there went the next 25 to 30 years.

Although Peter's isn't a sad or negative story but, rather, one of success, there are certainly aspects of it that warrant our attention, being, in hindsight, far from ideal and also showing behavioural traits to which many of us can relate.

In parallel with his professional wins, Peter also experienced several 'losses'. He'd lost touch with many of his old friends; he'd lost the involvement he'd previously had in social justice and politics (and with that, much of his passion); he'd lost physical health and fitness as time to exercise and play sports became increasingly hard to find; and ultimately, and possibly most sadly, Peter actually lost a big chunk from his relationships with his children. Quite simply, he just wasn't around enough to witness and enjoy their experiences with them—and do you remember those top five regrets of the dying?

Together, all of these losses help to explain Peter's 'terror' upon contemplating the end of his professional life, as it was at the time. For Peter, it was hard to imagine a life that didn't involve 60-plus hours of work each week; for Peter it was scary to imagine a life without the high levels of financial reward to which he'd become so used; for Peter, as much as he loved his wife and kids, it was highly anxiety provoking, imagining spending more time with people he barely knew!

As a relatively young father when Peter and I spoke, I swore I'd do my utmost to avoid this situation myself and have done the best I could to be actively involved in and present (as much as possible) in my children's lives. (Although I can't say I've come anywhere near to succeeding 100 per cent in this!) From a broader and more professional perspective, Peter's case serves as a stark reminder to us all that change is inevitable and that throughout life we need to be prepared to adapt and evolve and to redefine ourselves—preferably before change is forced upon us by some unexpected event or in an unpleasant or traumatic way, which makes it even tougher to deal with.

In response to a brief message I posted online, explaining a bit about this book and asking for expressions of interest from those who believed they could add something of value, I received the following simple response, which it seems relevant to repeat here.

Hi Tim,

I hope you are well. Happy to help out with your research if I am any use, my email is info AT allansparkes dot com, website www.allansparkes dot com

Best regards,

Al

As just noted, a simple response. Nevertheless, I couldn't help but think, *Who is Allan Sparkes?*

It didn't take me long at all to answer that question—and when I did, it didn't take me long to feel a range of emotions, including: a degree of ignorance and embarrassment that I didn't know who Allan was; a huge amount of inspiration just from reading about him and his experiences; and wonderfully grateful that he'd made contact with me and agreed to help out with my book.

So here's the short version of Allan's impressive biography taken, with his permission, from his website:

The Cross of Valour (CV) is Australia's highest bravery decoration and is also Australia's highest civilian honour. It is awarded for 'The most conspicuous courage in circumstances of extreme peril'. It has only been presented 5 times since the award's inception in 1975. Allan was awarded the Cross of Valour by the Governor General of Australia, Sir William Deane AC, KBE,

QC, for his rescue of a child who was trapped in a flooded storm water system in Coffs Harbour.

Allan has also been awarded some of the NSW Police and the Royal Humane Societies highest awards for bravery and service.

In December 2012, Allan was one of only 10 Australians to be awarded the Queen's Diamond Jubilee Medal, a personal gift from Her Majesty, Queen Elizabeth II. The medal was presented to Allan and 3 other Cross of Valour recipients by Her Excellency, The Governor General, Ms Quentin Bryce AC, CVO at a special ceremony at Government House, Canberra on December 14, 2012.

By reading Allan's Cross of Valour citation, you will understand some of what happened that day. It is a story of courage, determination and mateship. It is a story of how he and his partner, with nothing more than a torch and some rope, placed their lives in each other's hands to search for and ultimately locate and save a young child who had been swept 600 metres down a flooded storm water pipe. What should have been one of the greatest chapters in his life, quickly turned Allan's life upside down. Twenty years of front line police work had finally taken its toll.

Within weeks of Jai's rescue, Allan's life began a rapid downward spiral and despite his best attempts to overcome the demons that had taken up residence in his mind, suicide seemed the only alternative. The way Allan overcame this psychological crisis and the illnesses he developed is nothing short of inspirational. Since he was a young child living in the west of NSW, Allan's ambition was to one day sail across the oceans of the world and that is exactly what he did.

In March 2009, Allan and his family left Australia and boarded their yacht in England. Taking off on an adventure many dream about but few can contemplate, they eventually sailed nearly 30,000 kilometres back to their home port in Australia. Allan and his family achieved their goals with little true 'blue water' experience. It is an example of what can be done if you really set your mind to it, have the courage to believe in yourself and those who have their faith and trust in you. Allan's philosophy is a simple one; never give up on what you really want to achieve in this life.

Allan took on some new challenges when he came back to Australia, writing his biography, which was edited by Mark Whittaker, Walkely Award-winning journalist and award-winning author. A poignant story about Allan and his wife Deb recently appeared in the popular 'Two of Us' column of the *Good Weekend* Magazine, a feature of the *Sydney Morning Herald* and *The Age* newspapers. That story attracted the attention of one of Australia's major publishers.

Allan's book, *The Cost of Bravery*, was released by Penguin Books Australia on May 22, 2013.

As noted, this is just the 'short version' (Allan's full story is even more remarkable and requires a whole book to itself) so necessarily glosses over the extent and intensity of the pain and suffering Allan experienced. For me, as a clinical psychologist, it was clear after talking to Al that he suffered from what we call 'post-traumatic stress disorder' and 'major depressive disorder'. In simple terms, he had clearly been highly distressed and, sadly, suicidal and homicidal, making his eventual recovery all the more impressive.

However, none of this is why I wanted to include Allan's story in this book; rather, what struck me most about the man was his repeated reinvention of himself, his multiple redefinitions of who he was and how he wanted to live. Because it was doing this, I believe, that ultimately got him through the dark times and which is something that's so important for all of us to do throughout our lives, especially as we transition from 'middle age' into 'old age'.

So what were these different stages of Allan's life?

For many years Allan was a police officer. In fact, Allan was much more than a police officer—he was a passionate believer in what he (and his colleagues) were doing; police work wasn't just something he did, it was who he was. After being medically discharged (something that occurred against his wishes and something that exacerbated his distress and jeopardised his recovery), he retrained as a marine engineer and then specialised in marine investigations. Throughout this time he did several boating courses and, as told in his story, he then sailed his family across the world. More recently, Allan has become a writer, speaker and ambassador for Beyond Blue (an independent, not-for-profit organisation working to increase awareness and understanding of depression and anxiety in Australia and to reduce the associated stigma), not to mention the informal but extensive work he also does supporting other police officers who are struggling after having experienced similar traumas to those Allan experienced.

I'm not suggesting in any way that these transitions or redefinitions were easy for Allan. In fact, having spoken to him on a few occasions now and having heard him deliver an inspirational keynote presentation at a conference at which I was also speaking, I know most definitely that it was not easy, that it took time and that a wonderful spouse and several helpful professionals supported him throughout the whole process. But the key point here is that ultimately, Allan *did* do it—and if he could achieve it then so too can others.

Redefining one's identity has been shown to be of vital importance to those who go on to live healthy, happy and long lives. Allan is a remarkable example of that but even if the challenges you face and changes you want to make in your life are not as dramatic as they were from him (and I hope they won't be), it's still an issue to which we all need to give due consideration.

•

Before reading the research I reviewed so thoroughly for this book, if I'd been asked I would probably have noted that (psychological) maturation is not necessary; I might have added that it is almost certainly a better option than the alternative but, to borrow and adapt a metaphor, who am I to say that a butterfly is better than a caterpillar?

However, having read what I've read over the last year or so I have to acknowledge now that I was almost certainly wrong. Maturing psychologically might not be compulsory but it is, quite literally, a matter of life and death!

Referring once again to the Harvard Grant Study, one of the most interesting findings was that only four of the 31 men who failed to mature past Erikson's stage of Intimacy (young adulthood) were still alive at the 2011 follow-up analysis. Further, those who did develop to the Generative phase (middle adulthood) were three times more likely to be enjoying their lives at 85 when compared to those who still centred on themselves plus (and how's this for pretty amazing?) they lived approximately eight years longer!

Similarly, the Terman women (those from that other landmark longitudinal study into genetics), who failed to master what's technically referred to as 'generativity' (a concern for and desire to guide those that come after; a sense of optimism and hope for the next generation) were only one third as likely to report experiencing satisfactory physical intimacy in their relationships compared to others.

In the words of the ever-wise and poetic George Vaillant, 'There is a time for being a caterpillar, but it is brief.'

Looking a little more closely at this concept of 'maturation', it was interesting to see how the Grant men responded when asked to define 'wisdom'. At age 75, they typically said things like: 'Tolerance and a capacity to appreciate paradox'; 'A seamless integration of affect and cognition'; 'Self-awareness combined with an absence of self-absorption'; 'The capacity to hear what others say'.

Those who were not able to achieve this level of empathy and the balance between self and others were, if still alive, typically far less healthy and less well-adjusted.

Having seen that these findings reinforce the benefits of appropriate maturation, let's now look at one of the most widely used models of psychological growth—that developed by Erik Erikson, to which I briefly referred above.

In short, Erikson's model of psychosocial development includes eight stages through which a healthy individual should pass, beginning in infancy and ending in late adulthood. Each stage is characterised by challenges that (usually) people confront and master before moving on to the next stage. An inbuilt assumption is that unmet challenges or incomplete stages will contribute to problems that will surface at some later stage. It's important to emphasise, however, that individuals can progress to a new stage even if they've not fully mastered a previous stage, because advancement is not just dependent on successful accomplishment but is also influenced by biological, social and cultural forces.

Let's briefly review the eight stages of life, as viewed by Erikson:

1. 0–2 years—the key questions are around trust. Can I trust the world?
2. 2–4 years—the question shifts to one of autonomy and something like, 'Am I OK?' or 'Is it OK to be me?'
3. 4–5 years—we graduate to question what we can do and whether or not it's OK to do what we do (e.g. walk, move, act)
4. 6–12 years—the focus is on competency and we start to wonder if we can 'make it' in the world
5. 13–19 years—in adolescence the central concerns are around who we are, what we can possibly be and where we fit in with others
6. 20–24 years—we ask questions like, 'Can I love?' and 'Can I be loved?'
7. 25–64 years—the bulk of adulthood is about how we can make our lives count
8. 65 years-plus—Finally, during the age of 'wisdom', we tend more towards reflecting on our lives, questioning who we've actually been and whether or not that's been OK.

As you may well have already noticed, each stage includes a 'crisis' of sorts, whereby the individual is required to effectively choose from one of two conflicting forces, such as: trust versus mistrust; identity versus role confusion; and generativity versus stagnation.

It's these two final stages (generativity versus stagnation and pride versus despair) that I believe are most relevant in this book, but what do they really mean for those of us wanting to live a healthy and happy, long life?

Well, generativity, which occurs throughout 'mid-life', means that we're more concerned with (or at least are gradually becoming more concerned with) guiding and supporting those who come after us—the next generation. Anyone can do this by finding a way to work towards the improvement and betterment of our society.

One of the simplest ways we can achieve this is to support our children and help them set themselves up for better lives, but most experts in this area agree that real generativity goes beyond one's immediate family. It's one thing to support one's own children but it's another thing entirely to create something beyond family in ways that will ultimately prove beneficial. Those who fully achieve generativity tend also to contribute to other causes; they give, and they realise that giving can be done in several ways. We can give money or possessions, share experiences or expertise, give attention and love—we can even give or share knowledge and wisdom (which also touches on Erikson's final stage of development and maturation).

•

If, in addition to the maturation argument, you want or need more motivation to commit to giving time, then consider this—in giving we really do receive. Volunteers have been found to experience a range of psychological and physical benefits—something that's occasionally referred to as the 'helper's high'.

Numerous studies, many of which have included older people as their subjects, have found that volunteers live longer and enjoy substantially better mental and physical health in the process. It's possible that healthier individuals volunteer in the first place but the results of some of the studies are so significant and so profound that it's very hard, if not impossible, to dispute the benefits.

Consider, for example, the results of a study conducted on elderly volunteers living in or near San Francisco. Over a five-year period, the researchers found that those who volunteered enjoyed health outcomes 63 per cent better than those who didn't volunteer.

Part of the explanation for these impressive findings may well be found in other studies, which have concluded that people with stronger social ties and who have more and better relationships tend to report (and are assessed to have) better health as well as fewer illnesses than their less sociable counterparts. This discovery reinforces an enormous body of literature that has found positive relationships provide benefits in at least two ways—they provide more opportunities to enjoy positive life experiences and positive emotions plus they buffer against stress and illness.

•

In yet another of my favourite books, Stephen Post and Jill Neimark's *Why Good Things Happen to Good People*, the authors provide even more compelling arguments for the role of giving and nurturing other people's lives. In doing so, they refer, among other things, to the work of Columbia University psychologist Eva Midlarsky, who lists the following five reasons why we should find ways to help others and to give:

1. We gain a greater sense of the meaning of our lives.
2. We can cope with our own stress by shifting our focus onto others.
3. We feel socially integrated and connected.
4. We feel more competent and effective.
5. Nurturing others may lead to a more active lifestyle.

Based on my experiences, having worked with many individuals and spoken to and consulted hundreds of teams and organisations, I've developed the very strong opinion that there's no perfect or 'right' way to give; or at least there's no single way that's 'right' for everyone. So what's important here is to find a way that's 'right' for you.

When it comes to giving, give to something that's meaningful to and for you. If you care about the environment, for example, then find one of the many great organisations that work to preserve our natural heritage; if you love animals then donate to or get involved in the RSPCA, the World Wildlife Fund or Greenpeace or one of the other causes that prioritises wildlife and the animals with whom we share this world; if you really believe that we should do all we can for people first and foremost then do some research and partner up with a charity that helps children in the developing world or homeless people in your own city. As already noted, what's crucial here is that the cause and the organisation are important to you, because that means the returns you gain from your contributions of time or money will be far greater.

Mother Teresa was apparently once quoted as saying that, 'Not all of us can do great things, but we can all do small things with great love.' This is, I believe, a wonderful philosophy to guide this part of our lives.

However, maturation and development don't end with generativity. After and beyond this we come to the final stage of 'wisdom' in which we reflect on our lives and ask one of the biggest of big questions: is it OK to have been me?

The crux of the issue here is that it's not necessarily the person with 'the most' who 'wins' but, more so, it's the person who achieves 'integrity'. In this context this means that we've contemplated the sum total of our accomplishments and come to the conclusion that we've led a successful life because what we did mattered. Not surprisingly, those who see their lives as having lacked productivity or who feel they didn't achieve key life goals are likely to feel dissatisfied and even hopeless, helpless and depressed. On the other hand, those who believe they've done the best they could and achieved something of significance tend to feel more content and happy.

With all this in mind, complete the following simple steps to boost your levels of, firstly, generativity and then, secondly, wisdom and integrity:

- Reflect upon what's most important to and for you (is it people, children, animals, the environment, world peace, education, equality or something else entirely?). If you're not sure where to start, then have a chat to a few close friends or loved ones and ask them what they think you're most passionate about or, alternatively, search online for 'Australian charities' to find lists of charities and not-for-profit organisations, which will almost certainly give you a few ideas on which to reflect.

- Set aside some time to work out a 'budget' of time, money and resources; that is, how much money (if any) can you afford to give? How much time do you have that you could devote to the right cause (each day, week, month or year)? What resources or experiences or areas of expertise could be beneficial to others?
- Start doing some research and making some applications!

A word of caution here, because I've spoken to many (and even experienced this myself to some extent), who've found the process I've described above somewhat more complex than they'd imagined. (And even, in some cases, found it downright frustrating.) They think that just because they're ready to give, others will be ready to receive. But it's not, in reality, that simple. Even taking on volunteers requires resources (for supervision and organisation) and for some charities there's a limit to how many people they can take on and when they can use them. Many causes also have significant peaks and troughs throughout the year. (Think of, for example, the McGrath Foundation's signature 'High Teas' throughout October or R U OK? Day's national day of action in September.) So timing, preparation and planning in advance could well be vitally important when committing to charitable giving.

Further, for many charities where there's work involved with others, especially with children, there can be strict laws and regulations about who can do what with whom (which is, obviously, appropriate and necessary). The point I'm trying to make is that it's important to be realistic and not necessarily expect that your first port of call will be successful. Think of it like applying for a job; you might need to send off multiple applications and sit for many 'interviews' before the right opportunity becomes available at the right time. That being said, there are many great causes out there, desperately looking for great people, and so it's worth persevering to make it happen— a classic 'win-win' in which you gain all the pleasure and satisfaction of giving while the charity gains all your wisdom, experience and whatever other contributions you can make.

As for developing more wisdom and integrity, give some or all of these a try:

- To begin with, differentiate between wisdom and intelligence (whereas intelligence is what you know about life, wisdom is how you make sense of that information and what you do with it); the former has been found to be a positive predictor of successful ageing. (In fact, wisdom has been found in some studies to be more robustly linked to the wellbeing of older people than objective life circumstances such as physical health, financial wellbeing, and physical environment.)
- Take a few minutes to consider what one of the leading researchers in this area, Robert Sternberg, calls the Four Fallacies (which he argues 'intelligent' people are more susceptible to believe):
  1. The Egocentrism Fallacy—thinking the world revolves, or should revolve, around you (and therefore acting mostly

in ways that benefit yourself, regardless of how that might impact on others);

2. The Omniscience Fallacy—believing you know all there is to know (and, therefore, not listening as much as you could to others);

3. The Omnipotence Fallacy—believing that your intelligence somehow makes you better than others;

4. The Invulnerability Fallacy—believing you can do what you want and that you'll never come to trouble.

- Think of the wisest person you know (or even someone you don't know personally but about whom you've heard or read) and imagine how they live their life. Try to live as they would live—even if just for a day or two.

- Along similar lines, Jonathan Haidt (another highly regarded academic in this field) recommends reading classic works of literature and/or the writings and thoughts of great leaders and religious figures for inspiration and perspective.

- Make an effort to read news publications that are distinctly and overtly coming from a different political perspective from that with which you're most used.

- Use your experiences to help out family and/or friends—look for opportunities to help other people resolve disputes but think carefully before offering advice if you've not been asked for any.

- Set aside some time (at least an hour or so, if not more) to go back over your life in as much detail as possible and list any and all achievements you've made.

- Find some time to review your life with a few good friends and family members who've known you for a while; there's a good chance they'll remember and point out a few significant positive events that you've forgotten about or even discounted (we all do this a bit but it's not helpful to forget about or downplay our achievements).

• Make a real effort to fully think through and contemplate the implications of what you've done in the past; who did your actions impact upon and how might this in turn have impacted upon other people in their lives? (We often forget that we're all connected and so influencing one person in a positive way can then have positive effects upon other people in that person's life, creating a 'domino effect'.)

• Try to ensure your focus is on what you've achieved, rather than on what you've not achieved. Almost all of us will have some regrets as we get to the end stages of our life (as noted in the preceding chapter) and in many cases there are definitely benefits to confronting and resolving these issues, but this exercise here should be solely about focusing on the positives and highlighting the impact they had on our lives and the lives of others.

• Remember that 'wisdom' is one of the few positives that's frequently associated with ageing well, so make the most of this and all your relevant experiences.

• Reflect upon two or three key life choices and ask yourself, seriously, how you now feel about them. If there are any regrets, spend some time thinking about how you can come to terms with the decisions you made. (See Chapter Six.)

• Collaborate and discuss matters of importance with others. Research has found that 'social collaboration' (either by talking to oneself about what others might think or by talking to others about what they think) facilitates wisdom and wisdom-related performance.

- Write your life story. For Allan Sparkes, writing his autobiography was extremely distressing and difficult at times but it was also, in hindsight, extremely therapeutic. It allowed him to face up to and confront head-on several demons and, importantly, to redefine his story and to write it in a way that was helpful and constructive for him. There's much evidence to support the utility of writing and journaling and Allan's story is a great example of that.

When Allan Sparkes was medically discharged from the police force he told me he totally lost his 'sense of worth'. He described feeling as though his 'whole inner being had been sucked out'. He was aged 50 and for the first time in more than twenty years he was no longer a police officer. So, in his mind, who and what was he?

During our discussion Allan emotionally recalled how he knew he had to fill the 'terrible void' with something and that he was desperate and determined 'to become a better person than before'.

For Allan, his recreation came about from taking on a number of challenges, beginning with this epic sailing voyage around the world. This gave him, in his words, 'a new sense of purpose' and a completely new form of confidence. Knowing that he'd overcome both physical and psychological challenges provided him with a sense of regenerated strength and a belief that he could now do pretty much anything.

To cap it all off he explained how stunned and surprised (although, it should be noted, pleasantly surprised) he was when his story was so well-received—by the public, by his fellow police officers and even by the media (and then ultimately by the publishing industry). For Allan, this had nothing to do with fame or even fortune but much more so, with feeling validated.

'It meant a lot to me,' he said. Among other things, it meant, 'What happened was not a waste. I [sic] and my story could help people. And that felt good.'

What I've come to learn is that this process (which, for a growing group of people, is one that's initiated voluntarily or at least not prompted by an experience as dramatic as Allan's) actually has a name: it's being referred to as 'protirement'.

The notion of 'protirement' is relatively new and has replaced traditional beliefs about retirement (a word I keep trying not to use in this book, although it's difficult—if not impossible—to avoid it entirely!). The idea of working for one company for 45 years, retiring at 65 years of age with a gold watch, and then relaxing in a world of visiting grandchildren and playing golf seems to have dissipated for most. As technology improves and medical advances increase lifespan and 'healthy longevity', both men and women are living longer and having opportunities to explore and invest in more than one career in their lifetimes.

Protirement is the belief that, contrary to traditional views, retirement is as an opportunity to embark upon another career, pursue dreams previously put on hold, work for charitable causes and otherwise continue to exist as creative, productive members of another field. This, to me, seems to fit beautifully within the domain of positive ageing!

Exploring this idea further I found myself connecting with Alison Monroe of Sageco, a consultancy firm that specialises in career transition solutions; in simple terms they help individuals and organisations manage the changes that occur (or that they would like to occur) as people and workforces age.

Alison turned out to be incredibly passionate about her job and described a desire to help people 'work longer but differently'. She explained how this passion had grown out of a very personal experience, observing her father, who, after taking a voluntary redundancy aged only in his fifties, learned relatively quickly that the financial payout did not provide all that he needed to live a healthy and happy life. In fact, within a matter of months, he became bored and struggled to fill his days with meaningful and satisfying activities.

Alison's father, my client Peter about whom I wrote earlier in this chapter, and thousands upon thousands of others are coming to learn that 'retirement' is not what many of us thought it would be. Putting aside, just for a minute, the possible financial strains of maintaining a standard of living without a regular income, the key point about which I (and many others) am concerned is the psychological strain.

What will motivate you to get out of bed in the morning? From where will you gain your pleasure, interactions, daily structure or meaning?

Healthy and happy ageing requires planning in many areas of our lives including, as I hope this chapter has made clear, our careers. And even if 'career' no longer involves putting on a suit or dress and heading into an office to work for an employer, most (if not all) of us will benefit from having something in our lives to which we can look forward each day or week from which we'll gain and to which we can contribute.

This, again, brings us to the concept of protirement, but also highlights another area where there is, unfortunately, a significant absence of attention and effort.

Interestingly, the Australian government has partially begun to address this issue through its 'Corporate Champions' program. Via the Department of Education, Employment and Workplace Relations the program 'provides for a package of tailored one-on-one assistance to employers to recruit and retain mature-age workers (aged 45 years and over), and to promote better practice in employing mature-age people, and to provide a series of high-profile seminars and targeted communication activities'.

After interviewing many people and having begun to collaborate with many organisations on these and related issues, however, I've gained the distinct impression that most individuals and even many organisations are either not aware of this initiative or are not utilising it as well as they could.

That being said, the focus of this book is primarily on what you, the individual reader, can do to improve your own life and the good news (yet again) is that there's much you can do to take control of your career planning and to ensure that unlike Peter or Alison's father (or indeed so many others), you actively work towards creating a positive vocational path that will contribute to the positive and long life I'm sure you want to live.

The key phrase here is 'take control'. Of all the people I spoke to about the various aspects of this book, the notions of taking control and planning for ageing were constant themes. All of the health and wellbeing experts, for example, advocated taking action and starting as early as possible. Similarly, the research that supports the building and fostering of positive relationships (and there's much of it) highlights the benefits of beginning this in our early years. Not surprisingly, then, career or professional planning is also highly recommended by all who work in this area.

Unfortunately, however, very few people adequately plan for retirement in a constructive and useful way. The banking and financial services company HSBC recently conducted a survey of 16,000 people globally and found that four out of every ten Australians who took part had not prepared adequately, or at all, for retirement. That's 40 per cent of this population. (I was a little surprised by this, because in my experience the percentage of those who've not properly planned is much higher!) The survey also found that a significant proportion of retirees believed they'd retired too early and were not fully ready, either financially or in other ways.

This is a situation in which none of us should ever find ourselves. I've said it before and I'll say it again: just like in any other area of life, if you fail to plan you are, in effect, planning to fail. There are numerous resources available for those who want to utilise expert advice about financial planning, as there are, too, in related areas such as career planning.

Indeed, academics and writers the world over have proffered many models about how to do this, but Dan and Chip Heath (bestselling authors and professors at Stanford University and Duke University, respectively) have developed one of the simplest I've found in the process of researching this book.

The Heaths' model is packaged very nicely, using the acronym 'WRAP', which stands for:

W: Widen your alternatives

R: Reality-check your assumptions

A: Attain distance before deciding

P: Prepare to be wrong.

I particularly like the first two parts of this model. In 'widen your alternatives' the Heaths encourage people to think beyond all-or-nothing choices such as 'I'm working' or 'I'm not working'. They suggest that there are many options in between that warrant due consideration, and that part-time work and/or phased retirement is a workable and ideal option for many.

This leads to the second point about reality-checking our assumptions, which also relates to a number of the issues I raised in the first two chapters of this book. There are many myths and misconceptions about ageing, at least some of which will impact directly on our thoughts and beliefs about working and retirement. Consequently, many of our opinions about working may be unhelpful and possibly unrealistic. So consider carefully how you think about retirement—and, even then, prepare to be wrong!

At the risk of repeating myself, I'd like to reiterate the take-home message here, which is planning. Plan financially, plan professionally and vocationally, plan in every area of your life. You can always change your plans (in fact we often need to adjust and be flexible), but without them we're markedly more likely to end up lost and floundering, which is not at all conducive to positive ageing or living well!

JUST BEFORE CHAPTER EIGHT . . .

Having just spent the previous chapter focusing on growth and maturity it's worth reflecting for just a few minutes on what can be learned from the research and ideas summarised and on what's really the core driver of this important process.

Joshua Loth Liebman, who was an American rabbi and best-selling author of *Peace of Mind* (which spent more than a year at Number 1 on the *New York Times* Best Seller list), summed it up well when he wrote that, 'Maturity is achieved when a person postpones immediate pleasures for long-term values.' With this observation, Liebman implies that delayed gratification may well be important—which begs the question, how and why are some people able to 'postpone immediate pleasures'?

There are several ways this could be answered but all would have to include Liebman's 'long-term values'—or what could also be termed as a form of perspective. Put simply: what's it all about? Not just now, but the big picture?

These difficult and profound (but also important and necessary) questions and challenges lead us to consider themes that can variously be referred to under the headings of 'meaning' and 'purpose'. There's little doubt that those who have a clearer sense of meaning and purpose are more likely to live healthy and happy lives.

So come with me into Chapter Eight, where I invite you to contemplate these 'big questions' and where I hope to help you come closer to generating some answers and clarity in your own life.

CHAPTER 8

MEANING, PURPOSE AND SPIRITUALITY

'Man—a being in search of meaning.'

PLATO

I knew the name, the face and the reputation; I'd even tasted a number of her products. But I was still not entirely prepared for her positively infectious smile and laugh.

I met Maggie Beer several years ago, backstage at a National Conference in Brisbane. We were both speaking in the same session and so our paths crossed in the green room—the preparation area where we were getting ready and being plugged in to microphones and various other bits of necessary technical equipment.

For those who don't know, Maggie is a legend of the Australian food scene. She's best known for establishing (with her husband) the Pheasant Farm Restaurant in the famous South Australian wine-growing region, the Barossa Valley, in 1978. Her reputation, and that of her restaurant, grew off the back of her famous pheasant, and pheasant products such as liver pate, but she ultimately became even better known as a champion of locally sourced produce.

More recently, although Maggie has continued to operate a number of food-related businesses, her focus has shifted towards the production, selling and distribution of a range of gourmet foods, including the renowned Pheasant Farm Pate, quince paste, verjuice and a variety of spectacular-tasting ice creams (including my personal favourite, burnt fig, honeycomb and caramel!).

If that weren't enough, Maggie has also written a number of bestselling cookbooks and has appeared on several very well-received television shows.

And Maggie's efforts have not gone unnoticed. In 2001 she received the Centenary Medal for services to Australian Society through cooking and writing. In 2008 her book *Maggie's Harvest* won the Australian Publisher Association's Illustrated Book of the Year award. In 2010 she was recognised by the Australian government as Senior Australian of the Year and in 2012 she was appointed as a member of the Order of Australia (AM) in the Australia Day honours ceremony for 'service to the tourism and hospitality industries as a cook, restaurateur and author, and to the promotion of Australian produce and cuisine'.

At age 68, Maggie shows no signs of slowing down! But, as hinted at earlier, it was not her business acumen or success but rather her laugh and smile and obvious passion and enthusiasm that attracted me to her and which I remembered when I was drawing up my wish list of people to interview for this book. To have achieved what she'd achieved was one thing; but to be continuing to achieve with such zest and energy as she approached her seventies enticed me to discover what drove her and what we could all learn about living a full and vital life.

Unsurprisingly, Maggie was more than happy to talk to me about this book; the only problem was finding a time in her extremely busy schedule (which for me was a good thing because it meant she really was a living, breathing example of someone keeping active and ageing well). We did, eventually, find a time to connect and, as I'd suspected it would be, it was a thoroughly enjoyable and stimulating conversation.

Actually it turned out to be even better than I'd hoped. Whereas my initial goal was to discover what made Maggie tick, and how she maintained her activity levels, health and happiness, I discovered that she'd found a new cause to which she'd become devoted.

Extending the theme of food and good living, Maggie fervently spoke, for quite some time, about her latest projects on which she's working hard to improve the quality of food provided to those in aged care. She described being dismayed when she was challenged at a conference by someone claiming to be an expert in aged care, who argued that it didn't matter what patients or residents of care facilities were given to eat because they didn't know—and didn't care—what it was. The person even claimed that the nature of their food is less important for those with dementia because they won't remember what they ate five minutes after it's gone, anyway.

From Maggie's perspective, this person was completely missing the point. For her, food has always been not just something you eat for the calories or nutrients, but the very essence of life—food *is* life! And so to Maggie poor food means a poor life and, conversely, good food equates to a good life. And it is this philosophy that has effectively driven Maggie's life for the last four decades or so.

Although she was reluctant to go into details (and I had no desire or need to force the issue), she hinted at having had a difficult childhood. She briefly noted having had to leave school at the age of fourteen after her parents had 'lost everything'. But from this, she reports gaining her drive and resilience, her optimism and gratitude, providing a great example of the post-traumatic growth concept to which I referred earlier.

She repeatedly referred to being very 'lucky' to have grown up in 'the Valley' (the affectionate abbreviation used by locals to describe the beautiful Barossa region) and to having had the fortune of being surrounded by loving family and friends and community. Despite making reference to her family having lost much when she was only young, Maggie also told that having been 'given so much' by the Valley, she felt a desire to now 'give something back'.

The impression I gained from our conversation was that Maggie's many and impressive successes were never driven by a desire for headlines or attention or even for money but rather by a wish to improve the lives of others. For Maggie, as noted earlier, a good life is very much linked to a life filled with good food and so it was clear to me that her success has largely been fuelled by her ability to find ways to practise her passion.

And what impressed me even more was that she's continually reinvented herself and her business, modifying what she does and how she does it to take into account new passions and interests (such as her latest venture with aged care). Obviously, food and eating has always been a central theme, as has improving the lives of others, but she's applied this in many different ways and it is her ability to adapt and adjust that seems to have allowed her to maintain her energy, enthusiasm and passion over the course of so many years.

•

Maggie Beer is driven by purpose. Actually, it's probably more accurate to say that her purpose is what drives her life. This is important for all of us, but there's little doubt that it's one of the key factors that contributes to positive ageing. As noted earlier, when referring to those who live in the Blue Zones, having a reason to get out of bed in the morning is of vital importance.

And like everything in this book, I can make this statement with confidence because it's not just something I believe or even just something I've observed in my interviewees. I can make the claim that life purpose is important because it's also, crucially, supported by scientific research.

Midway through 2013 a Swedish study was published in which the investigators explored what factors differentiated 'very old men' from their younger 'old' counterparts. This interesting description was defined as those who were over 85 years of age (although more than half the men were over 90 years of age and a third were actually over 95). The men were all interviewed about various aspects of their experiences of becoming and of being 'very old'. The interviews were taped and then analysed.

Purpose in life was clearly identified as being an important factor for these men and in being described from different perspectives, enabled the researchers to categorise it into three main areas:

1. Purpose of life in general—this was mostly dominated by work, family and overcoming struggles.
2. One's own purpose in life—this was mostly focused on positive life experiences, making the most of life, recreational activities, adapting to change and happiness.

3. Reflections on purpose in life—which involved questioning the meaning of life and experiences involving negative perceptions from others about changes in and/or loss of physical functioning, but which was mostly about living an honourable life and being good to others.

Among other things, the authors concluded that healthy ageing was related to reflecting more on purpose in life, but especially reflecting *back* on purpose in life and planning forwards.

And life purpose doesn't just add to the quality of our lives, life purpose can also significantly reduce our risk of losing our lives! In 2009 the results of a collaboration between the Rush Alzheimer's Disease Centre and the Departments of Behavioural Sciences and Neurological Sciences at Rush University Medical Centre in Chicago were published.

In short, data from two different but related studies were combined and information from more than 1200 older people was analysed. The key objective was to assess the association between purpose in life and all causes of mortality in community-dwelling elderly persons (without dementia). What the investigators concluded was that greater purpose in life in life is associated with a reduced risk of all-cause mortality among community-dwelling older persons.

Both these studies, but especially the first when it refers to 'reflecting back on purpose in life and planning forwards' touch upon the role of an interesting concept that's often, in my opinion, undervalued; that of nostalgia.

Defined as 'a sentimental longing for the past, typically for a period or place with happy personal associations', nostalgia is often viewed in negative terms. In fact, it has, in the past, been considered a psychological disorder related to depression. But thanks largely to the work of Professor Constantine Sedikides, nostalgia is now being redefined—and it's being redefined in a very positive way. Sedikides' interest in this topic came about from some very personal experiences, when he moved from North Carolina in the USA to Southampton in the UK and found himself missing many aspects of his previous life. Rather than being made up of miserable memories, Sedikides describes how his nostalgia provided a texture to his life and gave him strength to move forward.

Reporting on this in the *New York Times*, John Tierney summarises Sedikides' research findings, noting, 'Nostalgia has been shown to counteract loneliness, boredom and anxiety. It makes people more generous to strangers and more tolerant of outsiders. Couples feel closer and look happier when they're sharing nostalgic memories. On cold days, or in cold rooms, people use nostalgia to literally feel warmer.'

He goes on to acknowledge that 'nostalgia does have its painful side—it's a bittersweet emotion—but the net effect is to make life seem more meaningful and death less frightening. When people speak wistfully of the past, they typically become more optimistic and inspired about the future.'

Interestingly, research by Sedikides and others has found that most people experience nostalgia at least once each week and nearly half the people surveyed in his studies experience it three to four times each week. What they refer to as 'nostalgising' doesn't always involve thinking about positive life experiences—in fact it often includes unpleasant thoughts and feelings of loneliness—but invariably people report that it makes them feel better.

'Nostalgic stories often start badly, with some kind of problem, but then they tend to end well, thanks to help from someone close to you,' Dr. Sedikides says. 'So you end up with a stronger feeling of belonging and affiliation, and you become more generous toward others.'

According to Dr Erica Hepper, another nostalgia researcher from the UK (the University of Surry in England), the usefulness of nostalgia seems to vary with age. She and her colleagues have found that nostalgia levels tend to be high among young adults, then dip in middle age and rise again during old age. Her findings, she claims, suggest that nostalgia helps people deal with transitions.

Dr Sedikides has gone a step further and considered how we can actively use nostalgia to build positive emotions and live better lives. He refers, for example, to a strategy he himself uses when he wants a psychological lift or some extra motivation. At these times he reports actively drawing on his 'nostalgic repository', by which he means focusing on selected memories and savouring them without comparing them with anything else.

•

Among his many and varied activities, Frank Dearn (that marathon-running marvel of 80-plus years) noted (almost in passing, towards the end of our chat) that in addition to running, continuing to practice the law and maintaining an interest in Rotary, he was also actively involved in his church. 'I have fairly strong [Catholic] Christian beliefs,' he said; 'and I'm an acolyte every second weekend.'

Generally, an acolyte (in the religious context) is anyone who performs ceremonial duties, such as lighting altar candles. For Frank, this has been an important part of his life, particularly in his later years, and although he wasn't entirely sure how, he believed this activity had contributed to his having led a long and healthy life.

As a psychologist, it's hard to ignore the importance of meaning—at all stages of life. What actually happens to us probably matters less that what it *means* when it happens and the nature of our relationships probably matters less than the meaning of our relationships. As discussed in Chapter Four, when reflecting upon optimism and gratitude, everything that happens in life can be interpreted in different ways and the meaning we ascribe to various events and occurrences significantly determines the quality of our living.

Numerous psychologists and psychiatrists have espoused this message, and I'll discuss this more below, but it also came through repeatedly when I was interviewing Australian television presenter and financial analyst Paul Clitheroe for this book.

I've been lucky enough to know Paul for close to a decade now and I say lucky because even though I've not known him all that well, nor been in contact with him all that frequently, I can honestly say every interaction I've ever had with him has been incredibly enjoyable and almost always fascinating.

For those of you who don't know Paul he's sometimes referred to as 'Mr Money'. This nickname came about because he hosted, for about ten years, a financial and investment TV program that aired on Channel Nine. It was, quite simply, called *Money*. This and other media opportunities came about because Paul was one of four founders of a very successful financial advisory firm, ipac, that he and his co-founders (including another friend and one-time mentor of mine, Arun Abey) established in 1983 and then eventually sold, almost two decades later, to AXA, who later sold it on to AMP.

Funnily, for someone who's spent the last 30 or more years of his life talking about money, Paul was at pains to emphasise (repeatedly reiterating during our discussion) to me that life's 'not about the money'. 'It's never about the money,' he reminded me over and over again. Rather, 'it's about what the money means to that person.'

Now some might think that this is an easy thing for someone with (reportedly) tens of millions of dollars in the bank to say and to some extent I'd agree. But knowing Paul even just a little I can honestly tell you that he believes this and lives his life accordingly.

From the very early days of ipac, it was clear that Paul and his co-founders were doing something they were truly passionate about. They had little or no money and in fact were only able to establish the advisory firm thanks to the use of their own savings and loans taken from parents.

According to the official history on the ipac website:

> They started out in a small room in a serviced office with just one telephone line. They had very little capital (around $100,000) and very few contacts.
>
> But according to Clitheroe they did have one advantage: a business they all believed in, based on quality advice with a fee for service.
>
> According to Abey [Arun Abey was one of the other

co-founders] getting their first clients was tough, and for many years the founders struggled, working long days and drawing only minimal salaries.

'We were 25 year olds, Paul was 27, with unkempt hair, talking to affluent, conservative 50 year olds' he says. 'No wonder my mother was worried'.

But they persevered because, as Abey explains, 'None of us could work in a job we did not believe in, irrespective of the money on offer.'

'With ipac, each of us was pursuing our calling. What we were doing fully engaged us and had meaning because we were helping other people.'

The fact they each went on to make a sizeable fortune was almost irrelevant to the hard-working and ambitious group; the impression I get (having met all four at some point in time) is that they're all more than comfortable with their financial positions but wealth was never the goal in and of itself. Rather, the goal was to do good and to help people.

When discussing some of these issues with Paul Clitheroe recently, many years after their considerable financial success and the sale of the business, I asked him why he keeps doing what he does. (That is, media work, books, consulting and speaking.)

His response was unequivocal. It's clearly not because he needs the money and it's because, quite simply, he loves what he does. He loves the idea of helping people gain control of their lives and he loves that he's in a position to help not just a handful of individuals but (due to his media profile and national reputation) the literally millions of people who watch him on TV, listen to his shows on the radio and read his books.

And this is what it's all about as far as Paul's concerned—taking control of life (specifically finances) by working out what money means and what (although he didn't directly use the word) happiness means.

In many ways, for Paul, everything boils down to meaning and purpose. And in many ways, based on my professional experience, research and reading over the years, I'd have to agree with him.

Meaning and purpose is vitally important when it comes to what you do and there's little doubt that the happiest and healthiest people I've met and worked with, at any age, have a much clearer sense of meaning and purpose than others. They know why they get out of bed in the morning and they know what they're going to do. They know what's important and, significantly, they also know *why* it's important.

Many times I've spoken to clients and audiences, who, for all intents and purposes, have been 'successful'. All of them knew quite well what they wanted to do and even how, where and when they were going to do it, but when it came to why, they really struggled.

And I don't blame them because I think this is a problem that's inherent in our society and it starts for many of us in our education. Most of us were raised (at school and at home) to focus predominately on goal attainment. We're encouraged to strive, to work hard to achieve and to accomplish and we're then rewarded and encouraged to set more goals and to work harder for more prizes. None of these aims are bad because we know that goal setting and goal achievement are good for us; they both make us feel good and are therefore an important part of happiness and health. But there is an important caveat; to get the most out of this behaviour our goals need to be meaningful—which is where the 'why' comes in.

This also extends beyond the day-to-day to incorporate much bigger and more significant questions such as:

- Who am I?
- Why am I here?
- What's the purpose of life?
- What does it all mean?

And if anyone continues along this path of questioning, they'll ultimately find themselves staring down the barrel of writings, discussions, attitudes and opinions about spirituality and religion; two enormous topics that warrant books of their own but about which I'll endeavour to offer a few useful thoughts and provide some practical guidelines as to how you can benefit from what the research tells us is important.

To begin with, let's read the World Health Organisation's (WHO) definition of what it calls 'active ageing'. According to WHO:

Active ageing is the process of optimizing opportunities for health, participation and security in order to enhance quality of life as people age. It applies to both individuals and population groups.

Active ageing allows people to realize their potential for physical, social, and mental well-being throughout the life course and to participate in society, while providing them with adequate protection, security and care when they need.

The word 'active' refers to continuing participation in social, economic, cultural, spiritual and civic affairs, not just the ability to be physically active or to participate in the labour force. Older people who retire from work, [are] ill or live with disabilities can remain active contributors to their families, peers, communities and nations. Active ageing aims to extend healthy life expectancy and quality of life for all people as they age.

So according to WHO, one cannot age positively or live well in the latter years without some degree of continued participation in spiritual affairs.

Dr Helen Lavretsky is a psychiatrist and Professor In-Residence in the Department of Psychiatry at UCLA. She recently published an article in the *Aging Health* journal, entitled 'Spirituality in Aging'. In this fascinating paper she thoroughly reviewed a range of issues, from the definitions of spirituality and health through to attitudes towards death and dying. Her starting premise was that 'interest in spirituality and aging has increased recently, owing to overwhelming evidence of positive health outcomes linked to spirituality and religious participation'. This is a bold and confident statement coming from an academic—academics usually being relatively cautious about making or even hinting at strong causal links.

But the evidence is there—and it is strong. Lavretsky refers to the findings from the (previously mentioned) McArthur Study and notes that evidence clearly supports a conclusion that 'spirituality and religious participation are highly correlated with positive successful aging, as much as diet, exercise, mental stimulation, self-efficacy and social connectedness.'

Not surprisingly, similar findings have been discovered in almost all populations, not just amongst the elderly. In a 2012 article published in the *Personality and Social Psychology Bulletin* by my friend, the sometimes controversial but always highly regarded Todd Kashdan (in collaboration with John Nezlek from the College of William and Mary, Williamsburg Virginia) from George Mason University, it's noted that 'to date, a considerable body of research has found positive relationships between the strength of people's spiritual beliefs and their psychological well-being.'

Spirituality is clearly important, then, and beneficial, but what exactly is it and how can we build more of it into our lives?

The first part of this question, the definitional aspect, is actually quite complicated and the cause of considerable debate. As noted by Lavretsky, 'despite centuries of debate, there is little consensus on the meanings and definitions of spirituality and religion.' That being said, she still provides us with the following common, and core, themes:

- a search for the sacred
- a search for the meaning of life
- a concern for the basic value around which all other values are focused (from the Spiritual Wellbeing Section of the 1971 White House Conference on Aging)
- evidence of spiritual wellbeing, including positive self-concepts, unselfish giving, moral character.

It's worth noting, as Lavretsky does, that 'spirituality differs somewhat from religion, which involves a more organised system of beliefs, practices, rituals and symbols, designed to facilitate closeness to the sacred and transcendent, and to foster religious communities. Spirituality encompasses religion but spreads beyond it to promote an understanding of the meaning of life, and an individual's relationship to the transcendent.'

I see little point, in this context, of debating too long and hard the definitions and differences. Rather, I think it's safe to say that one—the research supports the role of spirituality in positive ageing; two—we know much about the core aspects of spirituality; and so three—our focus should be mostly upon practices and behaviours that will enhance spirituality and, therefore, the quality of our lives.

Further, a fascinating publication co-authored by Michael F. Steger, one of the leading lights in the field of meaning research, revealed that although religious beliefs are important, what's probably more important is not 'what' you believe but 'how' you believe. (Michael is someone I consider myself very privileged to have befriended, having shared a speaking program at a national conference road show about happiness and its causes.)

By way of further explanation, the study supported other, earlier research, noting that one of the core psychological functions of religion is to provide meaning and purpose in life; but Michael's study also concluded that religious individuals will experience (and enjoy the benefits of) greater meaning if their religiosity is 'complex and mature, with an open, searching attitude toward the sacred.'

So what, then, can we do to become more spiritual? The following practices have been proven to enhance health outcomes and to improve the wellbeing and happiness of those who utilise them:

- *Prayer* and especially *group prayer* have been found to be very useful and are encouraged by pretty much all of the major religions. For those who have a traditional religious affiliation they will almost certainly also have some form of religious text (e.g. the Bible, the Old Testament, the Koran) that's considered holy and that can be read and followed for guidance. For those who do not have a religious affiliation, there are numerous alternatives that have been written by philosophers, spiritual leaders or even great poets and novelists. My only caveat (for this practice to be most effective) is that your choice of prayer or text is consistent with your needs (and even with your personality style), so choose something that fits and 'feels right' to you.

- *Meditation and mindfulness* have already been mentioned as strategies for building health and wellbeing but here I mention them again as paths to spirituality. The reasons they work have already been described but it's also worth noting that if spirituality is, at least in part, the ability to think and see beyond oneself, then the practice of mindfulness assists with this via the practice of (non-judgemental) observation and the practice of meditation can help by enhancing skills of clear and unbiased thinking.

- *Be open and curious* to new ideas and to new ways of thinking and believing. (This builds upon the just-cited research of Michael F. Steger and colleagues.) If spirituality is to be believed as a path, process or way of developing (i.e. the metaphorical journey as opposed to a specific destination) then learning is key. In another (2009) publication by Todd Kashdan (this time written with Patrick McKnight), three pathways to finding life purpose are described as: one—'proactive', which involves conscious and active effort over time, such as reading and attending courses or lectures; two—'reactive', which typically follows a significant, life-changing event; and three—'social learning', whereby we observe others—role models and heroes—and learn what we can through talking to or reading about them (e.g. in autobiographies).

I shall conclude this chapter, then, with the following recommendation—give some thought to the notion that spirituality (in a form that you can relate to) is good for health and wellbeing and then set aside time to practise your chosen form of spirituality, and the behaviours and ways of living and thinking it advocates, as often as possible.

CHAPTER EIGHT AND A BIT . . . .

If spirituality (including religion) concerns itself with the answers to life it is therefore probable that all the major religious beliefs and schools of spiritual thought have, in one way or another, concerned themselves with the big question of what comes after life.

As just noted in the previous chapter, there's widespread belief—even in the scientific community—that religion and its beliefs (or having a certain amount of spiritual awareness) are almost certainly good for us (because they're correlated with better health and more happiness). There's not necessarily agreement as to why religion, specifically, is good—and there are certainly a number of different hypotheses as to why this might be the case (as outlined briefly already)—but I'm going to suggest here that one thing religion offers us is comfort and reassurance about death and, perhaps more importantly, what might come after death.

In the following chapter I'll explain why it's so important to contemplate and to talk about death, because too many of us don't, which can perpetuate unhelpful and unnecessary fears and anxieties, which are not conducive to living a happy and full life.

CHAPTER 9

PREPARING FOR DEATH (SO YOU CAN FULLY LIVE LIFE)

'The fear of death follows from the fear of life. A man who lives fully is prepared to die at any time.'
MARK TWAIN

In a beautifully written and thought-provoking article by Sarah Macdonald in the *Sydney Morning Herald*'s Life & Style section, the heading 'Facing the end' is followed by the even better subheading 'We strive for a good life so why not a good death.'

Macdonald describes how, while travelling through India and Tibet, she trialled the Buddhist recommendation to meditate upon one's own death in the following simple, but poignant words:

I tried this while flirting with the faith in the Himalayas. I imagined a wrinkled, shrunken, incredibly old version of myself propped up in a bed and looking out to sea. I saw myself surrounded by grown-up children and gorgeous grandchildren. I felt myself loved, comforted and released. It was incredibly confronting. Yet it was also oddly comforting—helping me let go of a lot of my fear and loathing of death.

Macdonald then refers to how we prepare for birth (by reading books and by attending antenatal classes) and the fact that we prepare for many other stages of life as well—schooling, university, job interviews and even marriage (through the process of dating). But too many of us don't prepare for death; in fact hardly any of us prepares for death. And as a result, as Macdonald notes, 'most Australians don't die the way they might choose.'

•

As I've already noted, in my professional life I spend a considerable amount of my time consulting to organisations about culture, engagement, people-management issues and, ultimately, productivity and profitability. I have therefore read one of the most often-cited business books of recent times—Jim Collins's *Good to Great: Why Some Companies Make the Leap . . . and Others Don't.*

Good to Great is a fascinating story, based on an enormous amount of research data collected over many years, all essentially focused on answering one big question—what is it that separates those companies and businesses that have been and remain 'good' versus those that start off good and go on to be 'great'?

Here and now is not the time or place to attempt to sum up the many fascinating findings of Collins and his team, but I'd like to share with you one story from their book that I believe to be particularly relevant to this chapter.

Among the many factors Jim Collins explored to determine whether or not they were vital contributors to 'greatness' was, not all that surprisingly, leadership. And in exploring the issue of leadership he met with and interviewed a number of leaders in the field, including Admiral Jim Stockdale.

At the time they met, Stockdale was an academic at the Hoover Institute, part of Stanford University, studying stoic philosophers. In a previous life, however, he'd been the highest ranking US military officer in what came to be known as the Hanoi Hilton (a notorious prisoner-of-war camp in Vietnam). After having been shot down he spent eight years there, imprisoned in atrocious conditions, without any rights or set release date or any certainty at all that he would ever see his family and loved ones again. On top of all this, as the senior ranking officer he also shouldered a significant amount of the responsibility for his fellow prisoners. Incredibly, despite physical and psychological torture, and unimaginably tough conditions, Stockdale prevailed. But more than just prevailing himself, he helped his fellow soldiers prevail also.

How?

'I never lost faith in the end of the story', he's quoted as saying in *Good to Great*.

The reason I'm sharing this story here is not to highlight Stockdale's remarkable and inspirational resilience (although that would easily be a good enough reason to do so), but rather to show his approach to life, which was revealed in the book when he was asked by Jim Collins about why some *didn't make it out of the prisoner-of-war camp* (because unfortunately many didn't survive its horrors and deprivations).

Apparently without much thought, Stockdale answered, 'Oh, that's easy. The optimists.'

Jim Collins reports being confused by this response but I was completely stunned. As referred to in Chapter Four, we (psychologists) know from about 50 or 60 years of research and several hundred (possibly even several thousand) published academic research papers that optimism is, undoubtedly, a good thing to have and to use. Yet here was someone saying the optimists didn't make it out.

After I picked myself up from the floor I kept reading and, thankfully, it all began to make sense as Stockdale went on to explain his answer.

'Oh, they [the optimists] were the ones who said, "We're going to be out by Christmas." And Christmas would come, and Christmas could go. Then they'd say, "We're going to be out by Easter." And Easter would come, and Easter would go. And then Thanksgiving, and then it would be Christmas again. And they died of a broken heart.'

He went on to explain even further. 'This is a very important lesson. You must never confuse faith that you will prevail in the end—which you can never afford to lose—with the discipline to confront the most brutal facts of your current reality, whatever they might be.'

So in my language it wasn't so much the 'optimists' that didn't survive as the 'un-realists', those who continually set unrealistic goals and held unrealistic expectations, setting themselves up for failure over and over again and, ultimately, crumbling under the pressure of disappointment and hopelessness.

Those who did survive were what I would call 'real' optimists because real optimists maintain a hope in a positive future while also staying focused on the cold hard realities; and when they focus on the cold hard realities they focus on them in a constructive way. This is what the survivors did and this is what we all need to do to live a successful life—to be 'great'.

So what's the relevance here? Well, in short, the cold hard reality we all need to face at some point in our lives is death. As the saying goes, it's as inevitable as taxes!

Perhaps 'need' is too strong a word—many people go through their lives not facing up to this unavoidable certainty—but my premise is that in not facing up to death we rob ourselves of the ability to live a full and meaningful, happy and healthy life. As Jim Stockdale's experiences illustrate, a positive focus is important but not if coupled with denial.

•

On June 12, 2013, as I was in the very early stages of writing this book, I opened the Sunday papers to read the following:

By Tracey Spicer

Dear Mum,

I'm so sorry I didn't kill you.

I came close, believe me.

The pillow was millimetres from your mouth.

But I just couldn't do it.

How could I take life from the one who gave it to me?

My suckler and snuggler, role model and mentor, nurturer and nemesis: yes, you were all of those things.

To your daughters you were an impossible picture of perfection.

Successful career woman, devoted wife, loving mother—a feminist before your time. You laid out your manifesto: 'I want you to be independent women. You don't have to have babies. The world is your oyster. Go out there and show them what you're made of! Who says you have to be sugar and spice and all things nice?'

Brave, bold and beautiful, you always called a spade a bloody shovel.

Possessed of a wicked wit, you could cut to the quick.

That humour came in handy the day you were diagnosed.

The oncologist held up an x-ray, dappled with snowflakes (unusual, on a sunny day in March).

'You can see the cancer here, here, here . . . and here,' he said.

'It has spread from the pancreas to the lungs. Any chemotherapy will be palliative.'

You turned to Dad with a wry smile: 'Might as well go outside for a smoke. No point giving up now!'

I had to laugh.

At a family meeting that night, you were chairman of the board.

Speaking simply yet eloquently, you set KPIs for the coming months.

There was to be no pity, no moping, and no wailing: but there must be mercy.

A conversation we'd had many times around the dinner table suddenly had currency.

'If I lose control of my faculties then put me down,' you said, clearly.

'They do it to dogs. Why can't they do it with us, as well?'

We all agreed.

Voluntary euthanasia had never been up for debate in our house: it was a given.

The next six months were the worst—and best—of my life.

We looked at old photos, decorated with '70s flares, floppy sunhats and floral jumpsuits.

(Incidentally, why did you sew matching outfits for Suzie and me? We weren't even twins! I should have taken you to The Hague for those purple and green smocks. They were a crime against humanity.)

You gazed at me lovingly as I stabbed needles into your stomach, managed to keep down a modicum of meals, and patiently painted shadow boxes as precious keepsakes.

We laughed at the bandannas you made us to wear to your chemo sessions, at my dreadful Manuel impressions in the kitchen, and at the stupid things people said when they dropped by.

'Oh, we know it's terminal. But it's a gift, isn't it? All this special time you'll be having together in these next few months,' they'd sigh.

Well, if that's a f---ing gift, I want a refund. It's clearly faulty.

One day, it all got too much. We could no longer care for you at home.

We drew up a roster so there was always someone to hold your hand during those bright sunny days and dark desperate nights.

Your screams of pain were blood-curdling.

It was a Tuesday, I think, when I pinned the oncologist to the wall.

'Is there nothing else you can do you for my mother's pain?' I pleaded. 'Can't you up the morphine to put her out of her misery?'

'If I do that, I'll lose my job. I'm sorry,' he answered, kindly.

We asked the nurses. 'Please, someone, anyone, end this godforsaken suffering.' (Which was a big call for an atheist: I had been forsaken long before this.)

They, too, were kind, patting us on the back saying, 'There, there. It won't be much longer now.'

It made me wonder—how long is too long?

Is there a mathematical equation for this?

'I've heard three shrieks, five hollers, and one 'Please, kill me now', is that enough, nurse?'

So we decided to do it ourselves.

Suzie stood there all night pressing that bloody red button to flood your body with morphine.

The next day she showed me the bruise on her thumb.

'I know I could go to jail but I don't care,' she declared.

But her bravery was for naught.

You kept breathing. And writhing. And screaming.

And so, at 3am, I got up from the recliner chair, lifting the pillow I had wedged behind my back.

I told you I loved you. And I lowered the pillow over your face.

It hovered there for what seemed like an eternity.

But in the end, I couldn't do it.

I was weak. A coward. Not my mother's daughter.

I collapsed on the floor, sobbing.

You must have known: you died hours later.

Finally, you were in peace.

Mum, I hope you forgive me.

Not for the clumsy way I've written this letter (you were always a masterful wordsmith) but for not having the courage to help you when you needed it most.

If it's any comfort, Dad, Suzie and I are campaigning for voluntary euthanasia.

This was my wake-up call.

Let your suffering—and that of so many others—be a lesson to those short-sighted, selfish, puerile politicians who refuse to show compassion to their fellow man. And woman.

How many of them have seen someone they love die in agony, and live with feelings of grief, regret, and helplessness?

Like I do.

Love you Mum.

Your daughter,

Tracey xxx

Reading the Sunday papers is usually a pretty relaxed and light-hearted affair, but as I wiped away a tear from the corner of my eye, all I could think was *Wow!* The powerful effect this article had on me was made all the more intense as I'd met Tracey a few times over the years—and because I'd had similar conversations with my own mother in recent years. (Although I'm very pleased to say that she is currently in good health and, thankfully, we've not had to come close to even contemplating the ultimate decision.)

I don't include this moving story with the intention of discussing the pros and cons of voluntary euthanasia—an incredibly complex issue in itself, that requires legal, moral, medical, ethical, religious and many other considerations. Rather, I include it here simply to start a conversation around thinking about death—not to cause distress or depression, but to foster a sense of control and, in a strange kind of way, happiness and wellbeing. (Remember Jim

Collins's Stockdale Paradox and the revelation that those who faced up to ugly truths and tough realities fared better?) I therefore include it not for death's sake, but for the sake of fully living!

•

Not surprisingly, most—if not all—religions have given considerable thought and attention to the issue of death. Perhaps most noticeable among them is Buddhism, as illustrated by Sarah Macdonald earlier in this chapter, whose believers are encouraged to actively meditate upon death, which is considered to be very important for Buddhists for at least two reasons.

Firstly, contemplating death highlights the impermanence of life and Buddhists consider that it's only by recognising how short life is that we can also recognise how precious it is. Following on from this, the assumption is that if we fully appreciate life we'll then be more likely to fully live life.

Secondly, Buddhists also believe that by understanding and familiarising oneself with death and the processes of death it then becomes possible—or at least far more likely—to remove fear from a time of life that can, for many people, be highly anxiety-provoking.

Buddhism is certainly not the only religion or form of spirituality that encourages coming to terms with death. In fact, all of the major belief systems share a similar philosophy, which is essentially that not facing death is, in itself, a form of death. By avoiding thoughts of death we create anxiety and fear that can, if allowed, slowly (or in some cases rapidly) eat away our ability to live well.

Buddhism has, however, promoted the practice more vocally than other religions, by preparing and teaching a number of specific meditations that encourage the practitioner to regularly focus on death, the process of death, and what might happen after death.

In researching other perspectives, I stumbled upon an interview with a Jewish rabbi, who, at the relatively young age of 39, faced this very question himself. Rabbi Ed Feinstein of Encino, California, was diagnosed with colon cancer. His prognosis was not great and he had a wife and three young children. He underwent surgery and then a year of chemotherapy. His response to treatment was good but then four years later the cancer returned and he was told that 80 per cent of people with a returning cancer die. To cut a long story short, he was one of the twenty per cent and at the time of his interview he'd been cancer-free for ten years.

Understandably, the news of his condition didn't initially fill him with joy but not surprisingly for someone in his position and with his training, he responded somewhat stoically and thoughtfully.

'It changes the way you read all the prayers,' he was quoted as saying in the *Jewish Journal* article I found. When he contemplated the question, Who will live and who will die? in one of his prayer books he noted coming to the realisation that the answer was 'Me'. But he then went on to understand it would also, eventually, be everyone—because life is finite and we are all mortal. Rather than allowing the frailty of human existence to depress him, Rabbi Feinstein found it actually enlivened him:

If you really want to know what the whole tradition is about, it's about choosing life.

There is a line dissecting humanity. On one side, where most people live, is a world where you worry about who is going to win on *American Idol* and *Dancing With the Stars*, and you get upset with traffic jams and slow service in restaurants.

Then, on the other side of the line, are all of us who know that life is short and finite and terribly, terribly fragile, and we've decided not to let those things upset us anymore. We deal with a whole different set of realities about what is important in life.

One of the more obvious ways in which religion might provide comfort is the belief in an afterlife. Christianity proffers some form of 'heaven' or 'resurrection' and afterlife, while Buddhists are reassured by, or at least left to contemplate, reincarnation. So in short, although this might sound oxymoronic, for those who adhere to certain belief systems, life does not end with death.

But for me, this is not the only way the great religions can be helpful here. From a psychological perspective, one of their most important recommendations is, quite simply, to meditate upon death—to think about death. Because in thinking about and facing up to something we can become less fearful of it.

•

As mentioned at the beginning of this chapter, for the last ten to fifteen years I have, in my professional life alone, performed various roles, one of which has been as a conference- and corporate speaker. In doing so, I'm pleased to say that I've been included in some fantastic programs, worked with some amazing organisations and shared the stage with some truly incredible people.

Some of these people have been famous and others deserved to be; some have been inspirational and others thought-provoking; some have become friends and others I've never see again.

One person who ticks pretty much every box (although, thankfully, not the one about never seeing them again) is Petrea King—well-known here in Australia, she is inspirational, stimulating, entertaining, educational and one of the nicest, most genuine and caring people I've ever met. After interviewing Petrea for this book, I actually concluded our conversation by asking her if we could talk for an hour every week, because every time I connect with her I leave feeling good about the world and good about myself. And I know for a fact that she has that impact on pretty much everyone with whom she comes into contact.

As a result, I've been privileged enough to know Petrea for almost a decade now but for those of you who are less familiar with her, here's her story in a nutshell.

Not long after the death (by suicide) of her brother at the age of only 32, Petrea was diagnosed with acute myeloid leukaemia and was not expected to live. Understandably distraught, she escaped to the other side of the world (spending most of her time in a monastery near Assisi in Italy) and devoted herself to meditation, a healthy diet and processing a number of recent traumas.

Thankfully, she survived and has gone on to share the lessons she learned (along with her training as a naturopath and herbalist, not to mention yoga- and meditation instructor) with thousands upon thousands of people who were suffering. In the early days, she helped those with life-threatening conditions and more recently she's been helping those experiencing a range of chronic health complaints and a variety of mental health problems.

Now in her early sixties, Petrea continues to deliver roughly 40 to 50 conference presentations each year and the organisation she established, the Quest for Life Foundation, hosts up to twenty retreats annually, providing a tranquil and healing venue for those who most need solace to take time out from their busy and often stressful lives to enjoy asylum (in the truest sense of the word).

You'll almost certainly sense that I admire Petrea in many ways. On a professional level she's been recognised time and time again for her wonderful work and contributions to society. She's received the Advance Australia Award, Citizen of the Year award and the Centenary Medal for her contribution to the community and has been nominated for Australian of the Year each year since 2003, as well as being a New South Wales finalist for Senior Australian of the Year in 2011. On a personal level, as already hinted at, I believe she's warm, caring, compassionate and completely and utterly altruistic.

However, there was already something about Petrea that I admired well before I'd met her in the 'real world'—and that is something I still admire, almost as much as anything else, to this day.

The very first time I met Petrea was when I was invited to be a member of a panel discussion as part of an awareness-raising event organised by The Smith Family. As I often do in these situations, I conduct some 'research' into my fellow panellists so I have at least some idea of the people with whom I'll be sharing the stage and what their expertise and experiences are. As I learned about Petrea and her work I was struck by the name of the foundation she'd established. This might seem like a simple and possibly even superficial thing, but there's a lot in a name.

Just stop for a minute and reflect upon the work that Petrea and her colleagues were doing and continue to do to this day. Although not everyone who comes to her is dying, many are; and the others are often suffering to the extent that they've considered dying.

So what does she call her organisation? Quest for Life!

I loved it then and I love it now, because what she was saying to all those who approached her is that where there's life there's hope; while you're breathing let's live; and let's live today as well as we can.

At the same time, however, there is something of a paradox within this inspirational message, as I discovered when talking to Petrea for this book. Although all of her work for several decades now (and indeed much of my own work over the last twenty years, including this very book) has predominately been focused on making the most of what we have to live the best we can, we realised when talking that we both believed very much in the importance of not just focusing on the positives but also, facing up to the cold hard realities of life. And one of the cold hard realities of life is that one day, it will end.

When Petrea was first diagnosed with leukaemia she, and everyone around her, believed she would not live for very much longer. Once the shock had eased a bit she told me that she came to a few profound realisations. One was that 'If I'm going to die then so be it, but until then I'm going to live my life well.' Another was that she had to get herself and her life organised for the sake of her children and family.

Although confronting—remember Petrea was only in her early thirties—she reflects back now and notes, calmly, that by preparing for death in all areas of life she felt 'freed up to live!'

When I thought of all the various clients with whom I've worked during my professional career, Petrea's descriptions of her experiences definitely rang true. Time and time again I'd found that those clients who were able to face up to their fears and anxieties, pains and problems were far more likely to cope and function better compared to those who chose avoidance and procrastination as coping strategies.

Thinking about this, I posed the following question to Petrea to see if her thoughts and experiences were similar to mine: 'Given that you and I and many others know that facing our fears is important and beneficial, what makes it so hard for people to contemplate and meditate upon death and dying?'

It didn't take long for Petrea to start reeling off a long list of very plausible hypotheses (hypotheses, I should note, that are based on years of experience with thousands of very real people), including the following fears:

- of the unknown—what happens in between now and death?
- about the process
- of pain and discomfort
- of loss of dignity and privacy
- of loss of control and of function and of independence (including the ability to communicate and make decisions)
- of having to accept and receive support
- of the extent to which all of the above will impact on others (especially loved ones).

Interestingly in Petrea's experience, many of these fears are never realised and if they are, then, consistent with what the research tells us, they only occur in the very late stages of life (the final six to twelve months). Although they are still reasonable fears, according to Petrea's personal and professional experiences, avoiding thinking about them does not provide any real benefit but actually exacerbates the associated distress.

This reminded me very much of what we know about anxiety generally, not just anxiety associated with death and dying. As I'm sure you're well aware, anxiety is a normal, human emotion. We all experience it at times and it's perfectly appropriate to experience it at times. But for some people it can become excessively distressing and disabling and, consequently, highly problematic.

There are various reasons why some people's anxiety goes beyond 'normal' and becomes 'abnormal' but it is often due to the way the individual has coped, or tried to cope, with their fears. As with any other problem, some attempts to cope can be deemed (often after the fact) to have been more or less helpful and one of the more commonly utilised, but least helpful, coping strategies when it comes to anxiety is avoidance.

If you're afraid of something then it makes perfect sense to avoid that situation or stimulus; and if you can't avoid the situation, and find yourself facing up to something you're very afraid of, then it also makes perfect sense to escape from that situation as quickly as possible. This is a completely understandable response but—and this is an important 'but'—it's also a completely ineffective response, especially in the long-term.

Essentially, what happens is that avoidance and/or escape helps in the short-term by delaying or reducing unpleasant emotions, but what we also know from several decades of research is that this also maintains and strengthens the anxiety, fear and associated problems in the long-term. Short-term gain for long-term pain!

The good news, however, is that there are more adaptive and effective coping strategies that work in the majority of cases, which means that most people who are afraid can learn to cope with the focus of their fear much better and, accordingly, enjoy more aspects of their lives.

How?

The simple answer is to face up to your fears. As the saying goes, if you fall off the horse, you need to get straight back on. Facing fears robs them (the fears) of their powers; confronting anxiety ultimately leads to the reduction of that very anxiety.

Admittedly, this is easier said than done. If it were easy then everyone would do it, no one would suffer anxiety disorders, and many psychologists would be unemployed! But it is possible and it's distinctly achievable if one understands the subtleties and complexities of what's technically called 'exposure therapy'.

Exposure therapy, as the name suggests, involves exposing oneself (more often than not in a graduated and controlled manner) to the very situation and/or stimulus (a trigger, cue or 'thing') about which one is afraid. And the good news is that hundreds (if not thousands) of studies have demonstrated this form of therapy's effectiveness in ultimately reducing anxiety and increasing confidence and sense of control. In this case, short-term pain leads to long-term gain.

Let me give you a real example. Lisa, an old client of mine, suffered from what we call 'social phobia'. More specifically, she was extremely afraid of speaking in public. Fear of public speaking is a very common fear—in fact, it's the most common example of social phobia. For years Lisa had been avoiding this, in various ways and with some degree of success, but ultimately she came to realise that it was markedly hampering her social- and, most notably, her professional life (being too afraid to speak up in team meetings and/or to make presentations to colleagues can be very limiting).

After conducting a thorough assessment of Lisa and then explaining the rationale for such an approach, we collaboratively set up a hierarchy of feared situations. That is, we developed a list of challenges—from the relatively easy to the extremely difficult—through which Lisa needed to work her way. Such a process is a bit like climbing up a ladder, one step at a time, so it should also be noted that she had my professional support, as well as the use of several helpful coping strategies (such as applied relaxation techniques and a range of realistic and helpful statements she could say to herself in various situations).

Lisa's graduated hierarchy of steps looked something like this:

- Reading out loud, just to me, within the context of a therapy session.
- Preparing a 'speech' to read out loud to me, in session.
- Attending a Toastmasters meeting, purely as an observer. (Toastmasters is an international, non-profit educational organisation that operates clubs all over the world for the purpose of helping members improve their communication, public speaking and leadership skills.)
- Introducing herself within a Toastmasters meeting in front of people she barely knew. (Note: talking in front of people she

knew, for example friends and colleagues, was much more anxiety-provoking for Lisa, as it is for most people, than presenting in front of strangers.)

- Preparing and giving a short speech at Toastmasters.
- Asking a simple, pre-prepared question within the context of a team meeting at work.
- Raising a real issue, at an appropriate time, in a team meeting at work.
- Volunteering to present to her colleagues about the progress of a project on which she was working.
- Entering a formal public-speaking competition.

Now each step in this hierarchy was progressively more challenging than the last, but each step also became more achievable as Lisa gained confidence from each preceding step. I'm pleased to say that after several months of very diligent work, Lisa actually went on to win the public-speaking championships in her state!

What does this have to do with this book? Well, it has a lot to do with confronting the anxieties associated with death and dying for many people. As already noted, many of us avoid thinking about death, and all the accompanying issues we imagine may well occur, and in doing so we're actually enhancing our anxiety. What this book is about is living our best possible lives, living longer and living well, and I wholeheartedly believe that we can't do this if we're experiencing undue levels of apprehension (even if we're not aware of it much of the time).

So here is my step-by-step guide for confronting death and all you fear comes along with it, in a constructive and controlled way:

- Identify exactly what it is that you're afraid of.
- To do this, ask yourself, 'When I reflect upon death and dying, what thoughts go through my mind? What does death mean to me? What do I imagine death and dying will be like?'
- The answer to these questions will probably include some or all of the fears to which I referred earlier but it's important to clarify and specify which of these (and any others) are really relevant to you. (E.g. are you afraid of pain, losing control, loss of dignity and/or privacy, dysfunction, inability to communicate or make decisions, the need to possibly accept support and assistance, the impact on family and friends.)
- Once you've identified your personal fears you can then break them down into component parts—be as specific as possible so you can then confront every part of each fear in turn.
- Develop a gradual hierarchy, along the lines of that described above for Lisa's fear of speaking, that you can work through at your own pace over coming days, weeks or months.
- And finally, don't ever forget that you can ask for help; it may well be very useful to talk this through with a professional (e.g. a clinical psychologist or your local doctor) or at the very least, with one or more of your closest family members or friends.

One other interesting point to make about confronting fears and the outcomes of exposure therapy is that for many clients—those with phobias and fears of, for example, spiders and snakes—the ultimate goal is to be able to live a life without undue distress or having to avoid situations. For these people, the goal is *not* necessarily to spend each and every day patting or cuddling tarantulas or vipers!

The end goal of exposure therapy in the context of the fear of death (from a psychologist's perspective) is autonomy; by which I mean that we're not necessarily aiming to feel happy about the approach of death but rather to be in a position where we're able to actively live life without an intense fear of it. And this will come at least partially from taking control and making certain plans (as I hope I've already made clear).

This is effectively what my friend and colleague, highly respected clinical psychologist and bestselling author, Dr Sarah Edelman told me when I interviewed her in her role as Vice-President of Dying with Dignity NSW. On their website Dying with Dignity state their position as follows:

> We believe that individuals should have the right to choose a peaceful death when suffering is un-relievable and death inevitable. At least 80% of Australians now want the option of this final freedom.

Whilst she fully supports this statement, when I spoke to Sarah about the organisation's perspective on voluntary euthanasia she repeatedly reinforced the importance of the one simple belief that underpins their message—that of autonomy and choice.

As I've considered and discussed this issue with people who spend even more time than me working in this complex area, I keep coming back to this basic but vitally important conclusion: we should all be able to choose what we think is right for us, and indeed actively be encouraged to do so. But we can only make this choice, properly and reasonably, if we give it adequate thought. And giving the issue adequate thought and attention requires, at least to some extent, facing up to death and all the decisions and issues that surround it.

•

In 1996 the American Geriatrics Society listed nine important factors for quality of care at the end of life. These were endorsed and subsequently adopted by more than 30 health care organisations, including (among others) the American Medical Association, the Academy of Psychosomatic Medicine, the American Academy of Hospice and Palliative Medicine, the American Board of Hospice and Palliative Medicine, the American College of Chest Physicians and the American Pain Society. Several years later the list was extended to include two additional factors, as can be seen below.

Clinical policy of care at the end of life and the professional practice it guides should:

1. respect the dignity of both patient and caregivers;
2. be sensitive to and respectful of the patient's and family's wishes;
3. use the most appropriate measures that are consistent with the patient's choices;
4. encompass alleviation of pain and other physical symptoms;
5. assess and manage psychological, social and spiritual/religious problems;
6. offer continuity (the patient should be able to continue being cared for, if desired, by his/her primary care and specialist providers);

7. provide access to any therapy which may realistically be expected to improve the patient's quality of life, including alternative or non-traditional treatments;

8. provide access to palliative care and hospice care;

9. respect the right to refuse treatment;

10. respect the physician's professional responsibility to discontinue some treatments when appropriate, with consideration for both patient and family preferences;

11. promote clinical and evidence-based research on providing care at the end of life.

Now this book is not specifically about the end of life; it's about living life fully at any age. But the reason I include these guidelines here is to reiterate my belief that if we want to fully live life with meaning and purpose and without fear (or at least with minimal fear and anxiety) then we ought to give some thought to how we'd like to die. Forewarned is forearmed; confronted is less confronting. This list can help us face up to a number of the key issues and, accordingly, guide us toward making some of the key decisions we want to make, ahead of time.

•

I'd like to conclude this chapter, then, with one final effort to encourage you to make plans for your final years, months, weeks and days. Too many people, it would seem, from my interviews and conversations during the course of researching this book, have the erroneous idea that death is something that just happens to us. Yes, for some it occurs suddenly and with very little, if any, warning, but this is just for some and those individuals form, by far and away, the significant minority.

For most of us, death is something that will come slowly and even predictably. For most of us there'll be plenty of notice and plenty of time. How we use that time is up to us and how we use that time will determine the quality of our death as individuals, not just for us, but also for all of those around us (such as family and friends).

I'd like to take this opportunity, therefore, to advocate a plan I discovered and immediately found useful and attractive (due, largely, to its simplicity). Proposed by Judy Macdonald Johnston and summed up beautifully and succinctly in her TED (conference) talk, it was entitled 'Prepare for a Good End of Life'. Macdonald Johnston's advice regarding preparation involves taking five clear steps:

1. Make a plan.
   a. If you can no longer make your own decisions, whom do you trust to make decisions for you?
   b. If you can no longer manage personal hygiene or feed yourself, what would be your preferences?
   c. What, if any, life-extending interventions do you want used *and* not used?
2. Recruit advocates.
   a. Who will speak for you publicly if/when you can no longer speak for yourself?
3. Be hospital-ready (by having a ready record of the following):
   a. What aspects of your medical history are important for health professionals to be aware of?

    b. Which ID and/or insurance documents are important and relevant?

    c. Do you have (or want to have) 'Do not resuscitate' or 'Power of Attorney for medical matters' documents that should be copied?

4. Choose a place and caregivers.

    a. If or when you need more care, where would you most like to live?

    b. What resources or facilities are most important to you?

5. Discuss last words.

    a. What do you most want to say to loved ones, family and friends?

    b. What would you most like to hear from loved ones, family and friends?

    c. When would be the best time to have these conversations?

Obviously, there are many, many more questions one could ponder and these are just a few of the numerous, important issues I invite you to consider. The aim of this section, though, is not to cover every single possibility but rather, at the very least, to encourage you to think about, talk about and plan to deal with—actively and constructively—something that we'll all need to deal with at some point in time.

DON'T STOP BECAUSE YOU'RE TIRED; KEEP GOING BECAUSE YOU'RE ALMOST THERE . . .

And we are almost there; 'there' being the final chapter of this book.

But I certainly hope that won't be 'the end' but more of a beginning.

As you've read the previous 70,000 or so words I hope you've been inspired and motivated, stimulated and educated; but I also hope you've taken some action and put at least some of the strategies I've proposed and ideas I've suggested into practice.

I'm so pleased you're reading this book but what would make me infinitely more happy is to think that you're now, as a result of my words, living a different, better, healthier and happier life!

To be able to do so is your gift for the taking.

But in order to accept this gift, reading is not enough; even thinking is not enough. For real and meaningful change to occur you'll need (as I'm sure you're aware) to make some changes to the way you think about life and to the way you do things in your life.

Chapter Ten, then—the final chapter in this book on positive ageing—pulls together some fascinating and important research to provide some practical tips for creating a context and environment that will support your positive efforts, as well as strategies and tools to ensure those efforts become reliable habits.

CHAPTER 10
CREATING A POSITIVE CONTEXT AND DAILY HAPPINESS HABITS

'If you can't add years to your life you can add life to your years.'

The Northern Beaches area of Sydney, including the internationally famous Manly Beach, is often referred to (especially by those who live there) as 'God's country'. People who are born there rarely leave what they simply call 'the peninsula'—even to visit friends for lunch!

And there's a pretty good reason for the residents of this part of Sydney to be settled rather than peripatetic; it is stunningly beautiful.

Some of the best coastline in Australia, if not the world (especially in terms of beaches accessible from a city), can be found between Manly and Pittwater's Palm Beach, which is why I was pretty happy to find myself driving up the main road in this northern part of my city to visit Oceangrove Seniors' Living Village.

I'd been encouraged to visit Oceangrove by a friend who'd done some work with its residents and who, on hearing about my new book, thought that this 'lifestyle village' could provide a fantastic example of the new generation of accommodation for

older people. On their way out are the institutionalised retirement-
and nursing homes of yesteryear and on their way in are modern
homes designed for independent living that also incorporate easy
access to support.

When I first made contact with the owners of Oceangrove, I
received a very positive response from Sarah Sutherland, the Chief
Finance Officer for the neighbouring Dee Why RSL club who
first took the idea for such a development to the board about ten
years previously and whose (long) list of responsibilities include
business development and the overseeing of the running of the
lifestyle village.

Sarah asked me to meet her at the main reception of the RSL
club, where her office was based. As I waited for her I quietly
observed the friendly man standing near the door, who was
greeting each and every person who entered the club by first
name with a warm familiarity I could not help but admire. My
first impressions were therefore very positive and were only
strengthened on meeting Sarah. After a short friendly greeting
in her still-strong (despite having lived in Australia for many
years) English accent, we began a tour of the facility, beginning
by taking the short walk from the club to the village. As we did
so, we must have passed twenty or thirty people and, just like
the man at the door of the RSL, Sarah, too, knew every single
one by name (and they, her) as well as each and every one of the
most pressing issues they were facing.

'How's your grandson?'

'How was your trip overseas?'

'Yes, let's go ahead with that proposal.'

'Sorry about the misunderstanding the other day.'

Each new person was met by Sarah with the warmth and familiarity of a family member or, at the very least, a neighbour. Each interaction was positive and meaningful and there was an indubitable sense of community and belonging that, again, I could only admire.

As we then wandered around the village such exchanges continued. When we sat down in one of the small meeting areas, the constant flow of human traffic around us encouraged even more interaction but did not, in any way, feel disruptive, nor did it disturb the general ambience of calm and tranquillity that seemed to pervade the village.

Everywhere there were people but everywhere there was quiet; everywhere there was activity but everywhere there was peace; everywhere there were small areas in which residents could sit and talk or engage in activities and everywhere there were views onto courtyards and gardens and beautifully crafted outdoor spaces awaiting visitors.

If this sounds too good to be true, please trust me that it is true; and if it sounds eerily like a scene out of *The Truman Show* (a movie in which 'reality' was actually a creation of a Messianic movie producer) then let me reassure you, it wasn't creepy at all. Rather, it all seemed totally natural and real, genuine and authentic.

It turns out that none of this occurred by chance. Sarah shared how she and the other founders of Oceangrove had specifically instructed their architects to avoid large open meeting areas and instead to include smaller, warmer and more intimate spaces. At the same time, however, it was important that most of the smaller spaces had the potential to open into other areas, inside and out, so that larger gatherings too could be accommodated. The meeting areas were therefore specifically designed to be located alongside the main thoroughfares to encourage interaction and discussion and to avoid isolation. In fact avoiding isolation is perhaps one of the greatest strengths of the village, not only in its internal layout but also in terms of its position more generally. It's situated within 50 metres of amenities, including a supermarket, cafes, a medical practice and pharmacy; it's within a few hundred metres of a stunningly beautiful beach; and it's right next door to the RSL club that offers numerous dining options and, just as importantly, a plethora of activities and societies to which all residents (as automatic members of the RSL club) are given access. On any one day, if we include the RSL activities as well as those independently organised by the village social club, there might be card games such as bridge, day trips to near or distant parts of Sydney, painting classes and much, much more.

I'm not exaggerating when I say that in spending about an hour with Sarah, her team and the residents, I saw only smiling and happy faces—and this shouldn't really be surprising as everything I witnessed at Oceangrove was entirely consistent with what the research suggests contributes to a positive, healing environment.

•

We all know that excessive unpleasant noise (such as traffic, building works or even very loud music) and/or excessive heat or cold can cause stress; environmental stress. In the most extreme case, we know that living in a war zone or somewhere where we're constantly under threat can be very harmful to our health and wellbeing. Environmental stress of any kind can contribute to health problems (such as lack of sleep, emotional distress and even illness) but how many of us think about the way our environment can impact on us in a positive way?

A few years ago my family and I went on a pilgrimage; not a religious one, necessarily, but one completed by literally millions of families from all over the world each and every year. We ventured to Disneyland in Anaheim, California!

Now as some of you would be well aware, the creators of Disneyland describe it as 'the happiest place on earth.' And do you know what? They're not far wrong.

Opponents of commercialism and capitalism and even idealism might have a few objections, and they might have some validity to their arguments, but from a positive perspective there's little doubt that those Californians, led by Walt Disney, definitely know what they're doing.

Having arrived relatively late in the evening and being tired after travelling for most of the day, we (my wife, our two children and I) headed straight to bed after a quick bite to eat. We woke the next morning with much excitement and headed out early to beat the crowds.

Walking to the main entrance of the park was not overly exciting. Everything, as expected, looked clean and tidy and the streets were lined with the types of shops and restaurants one would expect to see just outside Disneyland. As we approached, however, the walkway opened up and we were confronted with the much-photographed sign noting that Disneyland is, indeed, the happiest place on earth. Having already purchased our tickets as part of a package at the hotel we bypassed the small queue that was forming and went straight to the main entrance.

At first it looked pretty much like any other entrance we might walk through but on the other side, without exaggerating, the magic started; the kids' eyes lit up, we all smiled and everything was just as we'd imagined but somehow we were still surprised, still enchanted, still excited.

Although I didn't give it much thought at the time, with the benefit of hindsight (and more than just a little research), I'm now aware that none of this occurred by accident. That is, the creators of Disneyland, guided by Walt Disney himself all those decades ago, specifically set out to tantalise each and every one of the senses to maximise positive emotions and positive experiences. Every minute of time spent in the park and every last detail was scrutinised and carefully analysed to achieve the desired results.

To begin with, Disney and his 'imagineers' recognised that although surprise and excitement certainly lead to happiness and positive emotions, too much of either can be unsettling, which is why they also included in their park many elements designed to enhance feelings of comfort and familiarity.

The first thing you see when you walk through the main entrance of Disneyland is Main Street, the prototypical centre of a classic American small town. What's not to like about—and who wouldn't feel 'nice' seeing—the local train station, signage for the local realtor and dentist, as well as ice cream and fudge shops? The wonder of the Magic Kingdom is just ahead, and just within sight, but visitors are eased into their day with some good old-fashioned and idealised 'normality'.

You'll be OK here, the creators are implying. *Everything is going to be all right*, you're invited to think and feel. And the creators are, of course, correct. The theme parks are very carefully designed to calm nerves, quell any anxiety and then gradually build on that relief and hope with just the right amount of fun and fantasy.

Interestingly, nursing homes and retirement villages all over the world have begun to incorporate similar principles to those that have worked so well for the creators of (and visitors to) Disneyland. I wouldn't write about an experience at a fun park just for the sake of it but I'm including this anecdote here as it illustrates some very important lessons we can learn from when it comes to designing the environments in which we live in order to live our best possible lives.

Nursing homes, retirement- and lifestyle villages, as well as hospitals and all manner of other facilities, are increasingly recognising the important and powerful role space and setting can play on our health and wellbeing and there's no reason why this shouldn't be just as relevant to how we set up our own homes and specific rooms within our homes.

In 2009 Esther Sternberg published a fascinating book, *Healing Spaces: The Science of Place and Well-Being*. In several hundred pages the academic and writer with a medical degree (whose research speciality is brain-immune interactions and the effects of the brain's stress response on health) sums up with beautiful anecdotes and fascinating scientific studies spanning neuroscience and architecture how our surroundings can (and very much do) influence our health and wellness.

It is largely from Sternberg's book that I realised the power behind the design at Disneyland but more so, it's from Sternberg that I gained a greater understanding of the powerful forces that don't just lie within us but also, around us.

As a psychologist I've known for many years now that the context in which we find ourselves influences how we behave. One of the most famous psychological experiments, discussed by every psychology student, is the 1968 publication *Personality and Assessment* by Walter Mischel that highlighted what's come to be known as the 'person situation debate'.

Do we behave a certain way because we're a certain type of person? Or do we behave a certain way because the environment we're in influences our decisions and actions?

Just consider how you act when you're at work versus how you act when you're at home with just your immediate family; or if you're out with some very good friends; or if you're with some new acquaintances that you don't know very well at all.

It's actually normal to behave slightly differently in each of these settings. It would be somewhat odd and potentially even dysfunctional to behave exactly the same way in every different circumstance. We are who we are but we're also different at different times and in different places.

The reality is it's almost certain that contributions are made by both personality and context, but the latter is definitely more influential than many people think.

Reflect, for example, on the Blue Zones mentioned earlier— those areas of the world in which people and communities outperformed comparable communities when it came to measures of longevity and healthy ageing. It could be argued (in this context) that these communities are 'set up' to encourage certain healthy behaviours and attitudes that then contribute to residents experiencing significantly fewer health problems and, therefore, living significantly longer.

As with pretty much everything in life, there are positives and negatives associated with this phenomenon but Sternberg's treatise made me expand upon the possibilities associated with such a finding and, accordingly, gave me great hope for what might be possible in terms of how communities, homes, rooms and even gardens can be created and designed to maximise health and functioning.

This notion is a vitally important part of this final chapter so let's go back to what some consider to be the very beginning of the scientific interest in the relationship between place and health.

In 1984 Roger Ulrich, a psychologist who's become most famous for championing the causes of 'evidence-based design' and 'health design', conducted what he believed to be an investigation into 'common sense' but what's since come to be referred to as a landmark study, 'View through a window may influence recovery from surgery'.

Without going into all the details, he examined the hospital records of 46 patients, all of whose beds were near windows but half of whom looked out to a brick wall and half of whom looked out to a view, including trees and greenery. In all other respects (for example the nature of the operations, the nursing care and the rooms) conditions for both groups of patients were near identical and patients in the two groups were matched for variables such as age and sex.

A very experienced nurse, who was unaware of which scene was visible from which patients' windows, then extracted recovery data from the available records. Among other things, this information included length of hospitalisation, number and strength of analgesics (painkillers) used, treatments used for anxiety, and the presence (or lack thereof) of common, minor health complaints such as headaches and nausea.

The results proved to be very interesting. Patients with views of the trees spent significantly less time in hospital and when the nurses' hospital notes were analysed were found to have received more positive comments (such as 'in good spirits' and 'moving well') and significantly fewer negative comments (such as 'upset and crying' and 'needs much encouragement'). They also took significantly fewer (in terms of quantity) and less (in terms of strength) analgesic or pain medications and although the difference was small they had fewer post-surgical complications.

So all in all, the patients with the natural view fared much better than those with the monotonous, brick-wall view. There's some debate about why this happened (was it the view of nature, of the colour green, the variety or something else?) but there's no doubt that a benefit was definitely experienced by those looking at the trees. And so what we can conclude is that hospital views matter.

More broadly, a study that might go at least part way to explaining Ulrich's findings was conducted by doctors Yue, Vessel and Biederman from the Department of Psychology's Neuroscience Program at the University of Southern California. Publishing their results in 2006, they asked whether there might not be some aspect within the structure of a scene that could be inherently health-promoting via its impact on relaxation or stress. Building upon the ideas generated by Ulrich and, later, others, they asked whether a particular view could boost mood and impact (positively) on healing. In short, their answer was yes—and what they found was quite amazing.

Biederman and his colleagues were aware that there exists a pathway at the base of the brain that leads from the visual cortex to another part of the brain, known as the 'parahippocampal place area'. In simple terms this pathway takes the signals from the eye (where they are first received) to a deeper part of the brain where they are constructed into a meaningful scene. (Interestingly, the nerve cells along this pathway have a very high density of receptors for endorphins, morphine-like substances that occur naturally in the brain.)

Now here's the punch line; the team from the University of Southern California found that when people viewed scenes that were considered to be universally liked, such as trees and sunsets and beautiful panoramas, the nerve cells in this particular pathway became very active.

Why's this important? Because by becoming active the nerve cells released more 'natural' morphine and so those viewing the attractive scene experienced a form of 'high'.

In addition to pleasant views, natural light is almost certainly an important component of the benefits seen in Ulrich's and others' research. We've known for quite some time that extreme lack of sunlight can cause a condition in those who are susceptible known as Seasonal Affective Disorder (or SAD). SAD is very much like Major Depressive Disorder (the technical term for significant and ongoing mood disturbance) but it's characterised as occurring in individuals and contexts where there's a distinct lack of sun and summer. (So it's far more common in the northern hemisphere, where prolonged and extreme winters can deny residents of certain countries sunlight for months and months on end.)

The flip side of this is that light has been used to help treat people with depression and has been shown to affect the mood and health of people in a myriad of contexts, including offices and hospitals.

Several projects have been conducted that are reminiscent of Ulrich's landmark study. One, for example, compared two groups of depressed patients and their living environments (whether or not their rooms were bright and sunny or low in light). Those in the sunny rooms were found to have significantly shortened hospital stays. Supporting this were the findings of a systematic review, published in 2008, examining the 'efficacy of light therapy in non-seasonal depression'. After identifying and reviewing more than 60 relevant reports, the authors concluded, 'overall, bright light therapy is an excellent candidate for inclusion into the therapeutic inventory available for the treatment of non-seasonal depression.'

It's easy to apply this theory to other contexts. Why, for example, would the positive effect of light therapy be any different if one changed the situation from that of a hospital to a nursing home or retirement village? Or, for that matter, any other environment in which people live?

The point I'm trying to make is that we should definitely be trying to design those places where an element of healing and recovery is required with views of and interactions with nature, but I'd go further and suggest we apply the same theory to those living independently, in their own homes, doing what we can to make the outside visible and/or to bring some nature in.

Multiple studies have been conducted in multiple settings—including hospitals, offices and other workplaces—exploring the link between indoor plants and health, wellbeing and productivity.

Overall, although there have been some mixed findings, there's enough data to support the conclusion that plants in the workplace are healing and they boost productivity (even reducing sick leave). As always, there's not complete agreement about how or why this occurs, but at least one study proffers that it's most likely due to the perceived attractiveness of the room.

It's not just the visual environment that's important, though. The sounds that surround us also have the potential to impact, positively or negatively, on our health and wellbeing and in some cases, on our recovery and healing from illnesses.

In *Healing Spaces* Sternberg quotes Henry David Thoreau, who wrote, in *Walden*:

> I wish to hear the silence of the night, for the silence is something positive and to be heard . . . the silence rings. It is musical and thrills me.

Anyone that's ever visited a day spa or even seen the (not always accurate) portrayal of a meditation retreat in a Hollywood movie will be well aware that silence, or at least quiet and tranquillity, is part of any healthy regime. Yet many don't experience this in their daily lives.

Think, for a moment, about those places where we'd most want to experience healthy and healing surroundings—hospitals. The unfortunate reality, however, is that hospitals (and sadly also many nursing homes and care facilities) are anything but quiet and peaceful for much of the time. Some studies, for example, have found that noise levels in intensive care units ranged from 45–98 decibels when measures were taken of all the machinery operating, heels clattering on hard floors, voices talking (and in some cases shouting) and the clangs and clashes of equipment on metal trays and tabletops. And this can go on throughout the day and even all through the night. Is there anyone who would find this relaxing? Is there anyone who would find this comforting or conducive to healing and recovery?

I think not. And for those of you who are wondering, 95–98 decibels is comparable to a hand-drill or a jackhammer!

Even for those of us who don't live in hospitals or institutions, all manner of noises pervade our modern lives, including traffic for those living on or near busy roads, aeroplanes for those living under or near flight paths and neighbours, especially for those living in apartment blocks or inner-city, high-density housing.

The reality is that although existing in complete quiet may be desirable, it is rarely—if ever—possible to achieve. (Excluding for those of you who are planning to create a new home in a cave in the mountains of Tibet!) There is some good news, however. We don't need complete quiet to experience the benefits of calm and relaxation; all we need is to minimise extremely loud noises as best and as often as we can while maximising quiet and tranquillity, and utilising the power of certain types of music. That's right—music soothes not only the savage beast but even the civilised adult!

We've seen already that the visual environment can have a positive impact on mood and health; well so too can our auditory environment. As just noted, extremely unpleasant noise can have a deleterious effect but thankfully pleasant noise can have a positive effect.

More often than not we call pleasant noise music. And there's an abundance of research that indicates the right type of music (noting, of course, that what's considered to be pleasant music is subjective) can have a positive impact on our emotions (and, therefore, our health and wellbeing).

In 2004, in the highly regarded *Scientific American* magazine, Professor Norman Weinberger of the Center for the Neurobiology of Learning and Memory at the University of California, published a fascinating article entitled 'Music and the brain'. In it, he reviewed a wide range of research, most of which focused on the question 'What is the secret of music's strange power?'

Among other things, he concluded that the 'findings to date indicate that music has a biological basis and that the brain has a functional organisation for music. It seems fairly clear, even at this early stage of enquiry, that many brain regions participate in specific aspects of music processing, whether supporting perception (such as apprehending a melody) or evoking emotional reactions.'

It's this last point that interests me most and that I believe is most relevant here, particularly because it is backed up in another part of the article: 'music evokes pleasure . . . when they scanned the brains [of study participants] . . . they found that music activated some of the same reward systems that are stimulated by food, sex and addictive drugs.'

And in another study, music was found to be able to influence emotion in both positive and negative ways, depending (not all that surprisingly) on the choice of music. In what was a very clever design, the researchers carefully selected a silent movie that they showed to a number of volunteers, who were divided into three groups. One group saw the movie with no sound at all, another group saw it with a score that was specifically chosen to be 'stressful' and the final group saw the movie with a specially selected 'relaxing' musical accompaniment.

While watching the movie, all participants had their 'stress response' assessed via heart rate and skin conductance (a measure of sweating and arousal) monitors. The results showed that those who watched the movie with a stressful score experienced significantly greater signs of stress activation than those who heard no music at all, while those who heard the relaxing music actually showed its having had a calming effect on them.

So sound, and specifically music, can have an effect on our mood and even on our physiology. Other studies on hospital patients have even found that music can reduce pain intensity and consequently the use of opiate and other analgesic medications (by up to twenty per cent!). Surrounding ourselves with pleasant sounds and music, therefore, could easily have a positive impact on our health, wellbeing and, ultimately, on the length and quality of our lives.

•

It's important to keep in mind that these fascinating and vitally important findings about the power of the environment in which we live do not need to be considered as relevant only in a retirement village-, nursing home-, or hospital context. Quite the opposite, in fact—the reason I'm including the findings of these studies and referring to them here is because they illustrate the merits of certain behaviours that each and every one of us can emulate and put to good use within our own homes and local communities.

Just as I was close to completing the first draft of this book I was very pleased to read about a brilliant example of much of this in action, just a few kilometres away from where I live in Sydney.

The Waverton Hub was planning to launch in September 2013 and according to their website it was going to be:

> . . . an active ageing initiative seeking to make the community more age-friendly. It is a member-driven organisation being set up by local residents for Waverton, Wollstonecraft and nearby suburbs [on the lower North Shore of Sydney].
>
> Many Waverton and Wollstonecraft residents have been experiencing the benefits of participating in The Hub's taster events and activities over recent weeks. Now it is the time for residents to join as members to enable the benefits of the Hub to be sustained.
>
> The Hub warmly welcome your participation and hope that you will become a member so that you can continue to enjoy the many benefits that the early days of the Hub are demonstrating.

- *The fun of doing activities together, enjoying each other's company and giving and receiving help when we need it*
- *Strengthening our community by being active contributors to the wellbeing of ourselves and our neighbours*
- *Having the stimulation of learning new skills, including through participating in building the Hub*
- *Saving money when getting useful services (e.g. trades people, transport)*
- *The convenience of easy access to help; local services and activities at our doorstep*

- *By creating Australia's first Hub and helping to build a replicable model*

Imagine how pleased and excited I was to discover this while in the process of writing a book that argued for the adoption and integration of these very principles into as many communities and facilities as possible! I couldn't help but get in touch to learn more.

It turns out that there are hundreds of similar community-based 'hubs' in the United States and that Waverton Hub was partly modelled on one such place in Boston, set up for residents aged 50 or over. Beacon Hill Village was established in 1999 by a group of friends who were interested in and keen to determine their own futures. They wanted to continue living in their own homes, within the neighbourhood and city that they loved, but they also recognised they might, at some point, need some help to maintain independent living.

Not being overly keen on the more traditional solutions on offer (such as care facilities and nursing homes) the friends thought creatively as they determined to hold on to their freedom and the control they had—and wanted to continue to have—in their lives. On their website they note, 'We wanted to take care of ourselves rather than being "taken care of"'.

Ultimately they decided upon the following, taken from their mission statement:

We are a community of people in central Boston who prosper from directing our lives and creating our own future. We are trendsetters for a new generation of people over 50 and invite you to join us in this exciting venture.

From this idea evolved the grass-roots membership organisation that's begun to spread throughout the USA and now, beginning in Waverton, here in Australia. Waverton Hub has literally just begun but Beacon Hill already has more than 400 members, which makes it sustainable. Perhaps even more impressively, in recent years Beacon Hill has helped to spread the ideas and concepts that it's so successfully put into practice. Following hundreds of enquiries and requests its founders published (in 2006) a manual in which they openly share much of their experience and provide a framework for others to copy. There are now more than 70 'villages' around the USA and the network seems to be growing steadily. There is now even a 'Village to Village Network', which hubs and communities all over North America can use to connect with and learn from each other.

Another great example of what I'd consider to be a wonderfully positive community is the University of the Third Age or U3A. This is a worldwide organisation that was started in France in 1968. The concept was so successful and so popular that it rapidly spread throughout Europe, the UK and then in 1984 it landed in Australia. There are now over 100 U3A groups in Australia with more than 40,000 members!

According to their website:

Universities of the Third Age, or U3As as they are more often called, are voluntary, non-profit organisations, which aim to offer older people low-cost educational opportunities, which operate in a pleasant, supportive social setting. There are no formal entry requirements, no examinations and no 'awards'. U3As are basically self-help groups built on the premise that collectively older people have the skills and knowledge to provide learning opportunities (education) for themselves. After all, 'experts' of all kinds in all fields eventually retire! In fact the word 'university' in the title is used in its earliest sense—a community of scholars who get together to help each other in a learning/social experience. Most of the groups in Australia are community based, but there are several, mainly in the capital cities, which do have an affiliation with and receive support from their local University. The principles of self-help and mutual support are the cornerstone of the U3A movement.

'U3A Online' is the world-first virtual U3A operating exclusively online. A quick scan of the website reveals an amazing and fascinating array of courses on offer (from Australian History through to Religions of the World and including, also, courses on creative writing, astronomy and even the eating patterns of earlier peoples), but the reason I'm including this here is not so much because of the awesome educational and learning opportunities on offer, although they are very impressive, but more so because of a conversation I had with a friend recently during which she revealed her father was very involved in the University of the Third Age in his local area (several hours south of Sydney).

During a casual conversation, Kerry told me how her father's life essentially revolved around his lecturing for and the organisation of his local group of U3A. She didn't refer directly to teaching or even to learning in an academic way but more to the sense of community and connectedness he experienced due to his involvement. She referred to the sense of purpose it gave him, the *raison d'être* he gained from it every day and every week, the opportunity it provided for him to remain active and to contribute and, as much as anything, to the friends and colleagues he'd met and made throughout his years of involvement.

I've seen very similar benefits cited and heard similar stories from my father due to his involvement in Rotary International (an international service organisation whose stated purpose is to bring together business and professional leaders in order to provide humanitarian services, encourage high ethical standards in all vocations, and help build goodwill and peace in the world). I've also seen much of the same, in a slightly different way, in my mother as a result of her passion for and regular participation in bridge (ostensibly just a card game but in reality a source, for her, of physical and mental activity, socialising and community).

So what are the key lessons here?

In short, anyone can leverage off the wonderful work of the aforementioned researchers and the creators of the villages and hubs, anywhere and any time. The key is really in taking the initiative and in taking control, especially of the following crucial variables:

- Wherever you are, join or create a community or network (ideally of like-minded people.)
- Use that community or network to provide support and assistance, depending on what's appropriate and/or required. (It's worth reiterating here a point made earlier, which is that health and happiness can be gained from giving *and* receiving.)
- Work to set up your network or community in ways that allow people to receive support without shame or embarrassment as

well as give support, ideas, advice and expertise, easily and conveniently.

- Remember that a problem shared is a problem halved; and joy shared is happiness doubled.
- Learn from the efforts of others—as noted, there are groups who have already made this work in several cities around the world. A quick online search for 'Waverton Hub' or 'Beacon Hill Village' will allow you to access lots of information and resources and to learn from those who have already created inspirational communities and who are willing to share their knowledge and expertise.

Another key message here is that health and happiness do not occur in isolation. Although we can observe those who live longer better lives, outliving their contemporaries, and identify (as has been done in many of the studies mentioned in this book) their intentional behaviours it's also important to note that these impressive individuals and communities (such as the Blue Zones) do not exist in isolation. No man or woman is an island and no healthy old man or woman achieves what he or she does in a vacuum.

Instead, as exemplified by groups like those in Sardinia and Okinawa, groups of people who interact often influence each other. They adopt healthy (or in other cases, unhealthy) behaviours together. As noted by Dr Judd Allen and Marie-Josée Salvas Shaar in their article published on the *Positive Psychology News Daily* website, 'Their positive health practices have become integrated into their friends, family, work and community cultures such that the healthy choice is also "the way we do things around here."'

And this is something from which we can all learn and upon which we can all build. Borrowing again from Allen and Shaar's writings, it would be extremely helpful to put some or all of the following strategies into practice in our own lives:

- Identify and spend time with healthy influencers (those people in your network or community who engage in behaviours you want to engage more in, too).
- Spend some time redefining what you consider to be 'normal' in your life so that those behaviours that are more likely to enhance your health and happiness become 'just the way we do things around here.'
- Develop ways to challenge and fight against unhealthy behaviours while also rewarding and encouraging more healthy and positive ones.
- Celebrate the positive leaders within your group; highlight their achievements and encourage them to share what they do and how they do it.
- Recruit those who are succeeding in your community (i.e. those who are most active and engaged) to teach and instruct those who are struggling (e.g. the less healthy and functional or the more isolated).
- Commit, any way you can, to building a community that revels in and savours healthy habits while making unhealthy and inappropriate ones as difficult to engage in as possible.

•

I've already referred to Harvard's landmark Study of Adult Development, led by George Vaillant, which followed and measured (on a range of physical and psychological variables) several hundred participants over more than 80 years and to some of the study's stunning findings, but a few key conclusions drawn from the research bear repeating here.

Among other things, more than 80 per cent of the study participants lived past their eightieth birthdays compared to only 30 per cent of their non-Harvard-attending contemporaries. Just pause for a minute to reflect upon the size and significance of that outcome.

Now even if one takes into account the fact that the participants were chosen for the study because they were deemed to be 'sound in all regards', I believe there's a strong argument for stating that by engaging in the right sorts of behaviours a dedicated person can increase, by two or three times, his or her chances of living a long and healthy life.

Let's see, once again, what George Vaillant (the most recent of the study leaders) has to say on this (based on his thorough understanding of the research findings and implications): 'People really can change, and people really can grow. Childhood need be neither destiny nor doom.'

This might seem like an obvious point to make but the unfortunate reality is that many people are what I'd call 'trait theorists'. That is, they believe that they are a certain way and will always remain that way. Even more unfortunate is that this view is reinforced by many who would appear to be experts—even in some recent developmental psychology texts it's been claimed that people, basically, change very little!

The Harvard Grant study and many others dispute this, however, and they dispute it quite strongly. People can and do change and although I could present you with even more research findings to add to those I've already cited, I think it might be more powerful to quote George Vaillant once again. In his chapter on 'maturation' in *Triumphs of Experience* he eloquently stated, 'it's true than an oak tree's leaves don't vary much as the tree ages—their shape and character are inherent fixed traits. But that doesn't mean that the tree itself remains the same. On the contrary, the grandeur and complexity of a well-growing oak do develop with age, enhanced increasingly by time and circumstances . . . The colour of the wine in a bottle of Chateau Margaux doesn't change much as the years pass either—but its character sure does, and so does its price.'

In short, it's distinctly possible to live longer and to live better by engaging in lifestyle behaviours that have been proven to be important; and notably, as already written several times, it's never too late to start making these lifestyle changes.

Hopefully I've also made clear in this book what these behaviours are and why they're important. But what I'd like to do now, in this final section of this final chapter, is summarise the key behaviours once more, along with some practical tips to ensure you know how to apply and integrate them into your daily life.

Let me begin with some wise words of advice from someone I've already quoted on a number of occasions; Frank Dearn, the marvellous marathon runner. When I asked Frank what kept him motivated and what, if anything, he said to motivate himself at four o'clock in the morning when training for yet another event, he responded with that most famous of quotes associated with that most famous of brands, 'I just do it.'

'You get out of life what you put in', he added, and you can't do much of anything at all if you're not fit and healthy.

For Frank, exercise was a non-negotiable part of daily life and although not everyone wants to run marathons this attitude is something I'd recommend everyone adopt. If you find something that works for you, a behaviour that will enhance your health and wellbeing and happiness, then make it non-negotiable. Just do it. As Frank notes, once you have to talk to yourself there are too many opportunities to talk yourself out of doing something!

•

Elaborating on this important idea, I'd like to spend the remainder of this book providing you with some tips that I hope will increase the chances that you'll be in a strong position to make it all happen. I've included in each chapter a number of practical tips, at least some of which I hope have resonated with you and appeared sensible and achievable.

I understand, though, that it's one thing to read about these ideas—and even to give some thought to practical applications and tips—but that it's another thing entirely to put them into practice in your life and then to keep them in your life, in the real world, day after day and year after year.

I was brought up being told it was the thought that counts and I suspect many of you reading this were too, but I'm afraid to say this is only half right; thoughts *do* count (as I hope I explained in the section on optimism and attitude in Chapter Four), but it's important to note that actions speak louder than words. You can have the best intentions in the world but if you don't do anything with or about them you'll never enjoy real and meaningful success. For example, you'll never get fit and strong without exercise (no matter how much or for how long you think about it); you'll never lose weight without dietary changes and you'll never enjoy happiness without the full and real utilisation of strategies and activities such as those developed by positive psychologists over recent decades.

So, without further ado, this final section will focus on how you can take what you've read about here, put it into practice in your life and, most importantly, turn what you start to do into behaviours you'll continue to do—the greatest gift you could ever give yourself: non-negotiable health and happiness habits!

There are, quite literally, thousands of research papers, articles and books written on the topic of creating, developing or breaking habits. I'll endeavour to sum up the key methods here but mostly I'd like to focus on and outline one of the simplest and most 'user-friendly' models I've discovered in recent years.

This model was proposed by Charles Duhigg in his book *The Power of Habit: Why We Do what We Do in Life and Business*. Duhigg doesn't offer anything radically or fundamentally new in this book but he captures, as many successful authors before him have done, the essence of what really works, presenting it in a way that's almost impossible not to 'get' and, just as importantly, a way that's almost impossible not to be able to implement.

So what is this model? Quite simply, it involves taking the following four steps:

1. Identify the routine.
2. Experiment with rewards.

3. Isolate the cue.

4. Have a plan.

Allow me to explain this a bit more, shifting the focus slightly to encourage you to use Duhigg's principles to create positive habits, rather than just focusing on dealing with the bad ones (which, although important and at times necessary to do, is not the objective of this book).

Why? Because the exciting science of positive psychology—along with many of the more contemporary studies from motivation research, self-determination theory and other areas of psychology and health research—strongly supports the notion that it's more effective to work towards things you want ('approach goals') than to move away from things you don't want ('avoidance goals').

So let's begin.

Duhigg refers to what researchers from the famed Massachusetts Institute of Technology (MIT) have identified as a three-part loop that's at the heart of every habit:

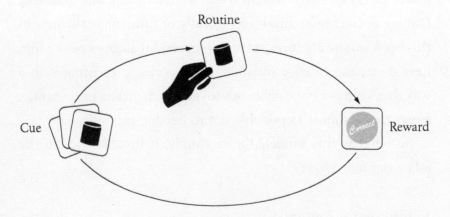

Eugene's Habit Loop

What this means is that every habit, good and bad, consists of a similar routine. Now over the course of this book I've suggested a range of positive strategies, such as thinking optimistically, exercising regularly, eating minimally and healthily and more. The challenge here is to turn these tips into regular habits and the principal I'm proposing is that this can be achieved by creating the right sort of self-perpetuating loop.

Let's, for example, start with exercise as 'the routine'. To begin with I recommend you clarify exactly what types of exercise are relevant and attractive to you and exactly how, where and when it would suit you to engage in it. When you've determined this, you've effectively taken Duhigg's first step—identifying the routine.

As noted, step two is all about experimenting with rewards. One of the strongest findings—across all fields of psychology, dating back at least 50 or 60 years and supported by literally thousands of research papers—is the notion that positively reinforcing (or rewarding) desirable behaviours is effective. Reinforcement, when utilised effectively, can increase the strength, intensity and frequency of relevant behaviours. That is, if a particular behaviour or action is followed by consequences deemed by that individual to be positive, desirable or attractive in some way, then that behaviour is far more likely to occur again in the future. A crucial point behind Duhigg's recommendation to 'experiment with rewards' is that a positive reinforcement can only be defined as such after its occurrence. That is, a reinforcer is only a reinforcer if it's been proven to increase the frequency of the associated behaviour. And here's the most difficult aspect of this point: different things work differently for different people and different consequences might even be differentially effective for the same person at different times of their life or in different contexts. This is why the notion of 'experimenting' is so important.

Let's go back to our exercise-routine example (although of course these principals can and should be applied to any and all behaviours and routines of interest). If you've identified what you want to be doing, along with where and when, then step two is all about providing yourself with some form of reward immediately after exercising, and then assessing its effects.

It's worth noting, here, that rewards can vary tremendously from person to person. They can be tangible, such as a favoured, post-workout (healthy) snack or putting a dollar into a savings jar with a view to eventually being able to buy something special for yourself, or they can be intangible, like the metaphorical 'pat on the back' or just a few quiet words to yourself, acknowledging how well you've done. Rewards can even take the form of something in between, such as monitoring progress and tracking gains to generate feel-good, positive emotions simply by reviewing a graph or table of improvements.

The most important outcome, which may well take days or weeks to properly determine, is that the desired behaviour(s) or routines are becoming stronger or easier to perform; this would be considered the hallmark of success. But that, my friends, is still not the end of the story.

Once you've identified the routine and the reward, step three involves understanding the cues; that is, what occurs just prior to the performing of the routine or behaviour. With bad habits, this is typically what triggers the unhelpful, automatic (and often unconscious) reflexive action or pattern. As we're focusing more here on building positive habits the cue is something you can create in order to propel you towards and/or remind you to engage in your healthy and positive routine.

On this point, Duhigg quite rightly notes that it's difficult to accurately identify cues because there are so many options from which to choose that many of us just feel overwhelmed when we try to reflect upon the pertinent ones. He goes on to state, however, that we can ease this stress by narrowing our search to five key areas, shown to be the most powerful and important:

- location
- time
- emotional state
- other people
- an immediately preceding action.

Relating this to our specific example of exercising, let me provide a few possibilities for your consideration. I'll begin with a few linked questions to prompt your thoughts:

- Where's the best place to exercise?
- When's the best time of day (or week)?
- How would you most like to feel in order to maximise your chances of exercising?
- Is there anyone with whom exercising would be more likely or fun?
- What can you actually do to increase your chances of starting your exercise routine or getting yourself to the gym?

Everyone is different but here's a possible example of the features of an effective cue:

- I'm more likely to exercise in the gym because there are other people around and I find the environment motivating.
- I prefer to exercise first thing in the day because I've found that if I leave it until later I'm likely to get caught up in other things.
- I know I'm more likely to exercise if I'm feeling positive.
- I enjoy working out with Mike because he's encouraging and supportive.

So . . .

- First thing in the morning, every Monday, Wednesday and Friday, I'll put on my favourite music to boost my mood and have an agreement to meet Mike on the corner of my street, from where we can easily get to the gym.

What we have now is a cue (or in reality a set or series of cues) that will trigger the desired routine that can then be followed by the chosen reward.

Duhigg's final step is to plan so that all the relevant pieces of the puzzle are in place and success is most likely to occur. If you can create, along these lines, positive plans using all the key strategies outlined in this book then I'm happy to say that I can pretty much guarantee you'll enjoy a healthy, happy and long life—including the very special gift that is the third age.

'Cease to inquire what the future has in store, and take as
a gift whatever the day brings forth.'
HORACE

RESOURCES

Websites/organisations
The Happiness Institute—www.thehappinessinstitute.com
The University of the Third Age—www.u3a.org.uk
https://www.facebook.com/LiveHappierLiveLonger
www.thehappinessdiet.com.au
www.twitter.com/drhappy
www.drhappy.com.au

INDEX